Wouldn't It Be Nice to **Have Someone**
on How to Consistently Get 80% of You
Highly Beneficial Treatment You're Rar

"Reserve Your FREE 30-Minute Team Training Call To Enable Your Patients to Achieve Better Health & Boost Your Revenue by $50,000 per RDH…"

Without Spending 1 More on Advertising

So Why Did We Give Up Offering Fluoride to Adults?

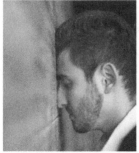

The reason most of our colleagues no longer offer Fluoride to adults is because we fear the inevitable response:

"Will My Insurance Cover That?"

The more I researched the rationale for giving Fluoride to adults, and the more I learned about the potential negative consequences of NOT giving Fluoride to adults, the more I realized I had an ethical responsibility to my adult patients when it came to Fluoride. I had a responsibility to ensure that I did everything ethically possible to make certain that they not only understood the need but were willing to accept the recommendation… even though they must pay out-of-pocket, because insurance won't cover Fluoride for adults.

The challenge therefore is that even though topical Fluoride treatment at the end of the prophy visit may be even MORE important for adults than it is for children, few know how to convey it to patients in a proven, effective manner.

Reserve your FREE 30-minute, live one-on-one team training phone call...

…and your team will discover how, in just seven sentences, you can achieve 80% (or better) acceptance of Fluoride by adults, who will gladly pay for the treatment out of pocket. Here are the results from just a few of the hundreds of hygienists who've gone through our 30-minute training:

Doctor	RDH	Adult Fluoride Paid Out-of-Pocket
Dr. Kirstin Ramsay	Suzanne	100%
Dr. Bill Gioia	Kim	100%
Dr. Michael Alsouss	Gabrielle	92%
&	Jamal	93%
Dr. Bob Dernick	Brandie	100%
Dr. David Hanle	Nicole	88%
Dr. Ike Lans	Michelle	90%
Dr. Anna Pollatos	Nancy	89%
Dr. Jerry Rinehart	Kim	100%

Reserve your FREE 30-Min. Live One-on-One Team Training Call TODAY!

Go to www.7SimpleSentences.com/BOOK5

WHAT OUR COLLEAGUES ARE SAYING ABOUT DR. TOM ORENT'S "GEMS"

"Hygiene profitability shot through the roof! Our practice is up a whopping $303,948!!"

—DR. JOE ALBERT, Edmonds, Washington

"It only took 90 minutes to implement our first Gem. In just 2 weeks we had a huge bump. Just one doc and a small team... thanks to Gems, in 10 months a $430,204 increase!"

—DR. TERRIE CRIBBS, Knoxville, Tennessee

"Tom, I have to say, without your help, I don't think we could have had the recent successes we have had. Practically a 50% increase for a one doctor, one hygienist practice in just 8 months. If I didn't actually DO it, I'd say it was impossible!"

—DR. KEITH KELLEY, Troy, Michigan

"My practice was already a comfortable one doctor private practice. In the last 30 months we've collected an extra $1,053,780.00 beyond our pre-Gems revenue... with more money in the bank now than I ever thought we'd have!"

—DR. JEFF COHEN, Covina, California

"Last year we collected $17,000,000.00. Recently a DSO offered me 8 figures (first digit *not* a one). I turned them down. With Tom's help I have built a dental machine that only needs about 15 hours a week, 3 weeks a month. I am living my pre-Gems dream!"

—DR. KELLY BROWN, Guthrie, Oklahoma

"Thank you for the best year of my life. Production doubled. In 10 months, my practice became something even in my wildest dreams, I never could have imagined possible."

—DR. BILL DONAHUE, Parkville, Missouri

"Of 80–100 hours CE we attend each year, none impacted our team and brought about renewed enthusiasm and growth as did Dr. Orent's Gems program."

—*DR. ROY HAMMOND, Provo, Utah*

"My practice was on its last legs. I think I was about 6 months away from just chucking dentistry at that point. With Gems, we had a $60,000 increase in 30 days and have nearly *doubled* the practice after just 4 years. Gems has improved my quality of life."

—*DR. ERNIE JERCINOVIC, Chicago, Illinois*

"It takes almost no extra time or effort, but the results speak for themselves! When I think back to the overall state of my practice (chaos) pre-Gems... how hard I was working and what I was earning (not enough)... all I can say is thank you, Gems! A 56% increase in our collections! You changed my family's outlook!"

—*DR. GINA JOHNSON-HIGGINS, Lexington, Kentucky*

"Less than a year with Tom and we're up $417,858! My team has become possessed!"

—*DR. JEFF BARTLETT, Fort Lauderdale, Florida*

"Tom's approach to team bonus is great. His strategies are really easy to implement. Gems has changed my life and reduced stress by helping us create a TEAM."

—*DR. KEVIN COLLINS, Metairie, Louisiana*

"THE most incredible year of my practice. Pankey I – V, LVI, AGD Fellowship, and Buchannan's Endo, some of the earlier highlights... but GEMS ROCKS! We were already a well-run extremely strong practice. Since joining Gems we're up $518,424 per year!"

—*DR. MARK HILDAHL, Minot, North Dakota*

"Gems made me more empowered to become the leader again of my practice and to take ownership. Before Gems, we were financially strapped. Since joining Gems, we will be up over $400,000.00 annualized by the end of this year!"

—*DR. MARY ANN GARCIA, Raynham, Massachusetts*

"Tom's ability to break things down into the real nuts and bolts has made the biggest impact on me. Gems has made my practice successful."

—*DR. STEVEN BELLORINI, Brewster, Massachusetts*

"In less than a year with Gems, I DOUBLED HYGIENE. My overall practice went up 70%"

—*DR. DAVID GRACE, Weymouth, Massachusetts*

"Following the economic crash, I experienced a sharp decline. It looked like my practice was just going to go down in flames. It was one of the worst periods of my life. Since Gems our patients are so much happier, my team is happy, and I'm just thrilled that the world has blossomed for us! We've nearly doubled our revenue!"

—*DR. SUSAN KLYBER, Berwyn, Illinois*

"Thanks to Gems, my staff is finally taking ownership of things. What I really like is even though I'm the doctor, Gems coaches speak to my staff and then without me having to drive it, they take a strategy and run with it. I've never experienced that before. My team is so enthusiastic! Heartfelt thanks from Barbados for our $454,698 increase!"

—*DR. ALLISON MAYER, Barbados*

"As a dentist and single mom, I'd all but given up hope of having any time to myself. Just 8 months with Gems and we're up $205,188. Thanks for helping one proud mom spend a little more time with her kids, less time at the office, and enjoy financial security!"

—*DR. BRIDGET BURRIS, Las Cruces, New Mexico*

"Dr. Orent's program has reduced my anxiety significantly to where I'm making much more money, yet I really don't feel I'm working quite as hard as I used to. We're now seeing 108 EXTRA new patients per year and have increased collections $831,036!"

—*DR. KEN RASBORNIK, Cleveland, North Carolina*

Transform Your
DENTAL PRACTICE
from
COALMINE to
GOLDMINE
BEFORE IT'S TOO LATE

ESSENTIAL GEMS FOR SUCCESS

Dr. Tom *"The Gems Guy"* Orent

CONTENTS

FOREWORD

We all have great days and down days in our practices, and some have long periods of frustration about the practice of dentistry. Tom shares his practice and life challenges with you in this book. He was determined to change! He describes his journey. The changes he made are possible for each of us. They transformed his life, and can change YOURS!

His "GEMS" can apply immediately to you and your patients and ultimately to your overall practice and your family. The optimism, enthusiasm, and positive thinking that accompanied his change are the "electricity" of life. We all need these characteristics.

Some of the topics Tom discusses in the book include the "Gems" philosophy and putting the "Gems" philosophy into practice, with lots of stories and examples. You will enjoy this real-world book, and it will increase your enjoyment of the recognized BEST profession as well as your practice revenue!

Gordon J. Christensen, DDS MSD PhD
CEO Clinicians Report Foundation and Practical Clinical Courses
Adjunct Professor University of Utah
Practicing Prosthodontist

HOW TO GET THE MOST OUT OF THIS BOOK, YOUR DENTAL PRACTICE, AND YOUR LIFE!

I hope you love dentistry. If you do, terrific. This book is for *you*. If not, one of my goals for this book is to help you reignite your passion for our profession. But no matter *how* much you love going to work every day, we've all heard the old adage... "Nobody on their death bed said they wished they'd spent just a little more time at the office!"

Dentistry can be fun, and professionally and financially very rewarding. However, dentistry is a means to an end. Ideally, the financial rewards from your practice should enable you to achieve AUTONOMY—the ability to work only *if* you want, with *whom* you want, and only *when* you want.

I achieved financial autonomy at age 46 and sold my practices. I now continue to work only because I love what I do, helping other dentists achieve *their* goals. This book contains several "Gems" and at least two epiphanies which I hope will help you move further along the path to achieving *your* goals—your dreams for your practice, yourself, and for your family.

Some of my goals in sharing this book with you are to help you help more of your patients accept your best recommendations for care, help them achieve optimal health and longevity... and as a result, **assist *you* in making more money in *less* time**.

1. **Mark it up!** Read with pen and/or highlighter in hand. Anytime you find a Gem you'd like to deploy in your practice, circle it, star it, write notes in the margins and/or dog-ear the bottom corner of the page so you can find it easily.

2. **Watch the FREE BONUS VIDEOS right away.**
Following several of the Gems I share in this book, I give
you a link to watch a FREE VIDEO TEAM TRAINING
TOOLKIT. Although there's more than enough detail right
within these pages to deploy several of my Gems in your
practice, taking advantage of the FREE VIDEOS will
ensure even faster, better results.

3. **Read, Encounter, Deploy, Repeat!** This isn't a novel!
Immediately upon encountering a Gem you like, put the
book down and *deploy* the Gem! There's nothing more
likely to help you achieve your highest success than taking
immediate action! Then after you've deployed the concept
and *proven* to yourself that Gems Are Easy, pick up the
book and continue reading where you left off.

4. **Make More Money in Less Time!** Sure, it sounds
impossible. But I can *assure* you it's not only possible but
being done by many of my Gems Family Members today. If
you follow steps 1 through 3 above, you'll be well on your
way to helping your patients achieve better health, making
more money for yourself and your family, and yes, spending
less time at the office as a result.

5. **Download the FREE AUDIOBOOK** As my way of
saying thanks, I would like to give you ABSOLUTELY FREE
as my gift to you, the AUDIO BOOK VERSION of *CoalMine
to GoldMine!* PLUS, a FREE VERBAL SKILLS TOOLKIT
proven to help patients to achieve better health and
increase your practice revenue by as much as $50,000!

   **Go to www.CoaltoGold.com/AUDIOBOOK to get
   your free gifts today!**

6. **Sign up for my FREE PODCAST:**
www.CoalmineToGoldmine.com Now you can *listen*
to Gems at the gym, on your bike, driving your car, or on a
long hike. Although I'm 6'2", through the magic technology

of podcasting now I'm as portable as your iPhone or Droid! Don't miss a single episode. Sign up today!

7. **Take a FREE 6-week Test Drive of my Gems Family Platinum Team Training Toolkit: www.GemsAreEasy.com/Book5**. You will get instant access to team trainings, ready-to-use marketing materials, and other Gems that could add hundreds of thousands of dollars to your bottom line.

Imagine what it would be like to be *living* the life of your dreams. Well, you need not imagine. With this book, Gems in hand, you've already taken a great first step towards *achieving* and living your dream.

Elizabeth and I would like to thank you for the opportunity to share the Gems with you.

Dr. Tom *"The Gems Guy"* Orent

OUR MISSION:

"Together we are dedicated to improving the health and longevity of 3,000,000 people, one smile at a time!"

INTRODUCTION

"HIDDEN PAIN, SECRET SHAME"

Too many dentists in private practice share a secret.

What is this embarrassing truth? They are unfulfilled—professionally and financially. They feel frustrated, prevented from providing patients with the high level of care they're trained to perform.

Not only that, many dentists are further away from financial independence than they should be. They have nothing—or at least far too little—put away for retirement.

Others are doing well, but they've plateaued. They'd love to build their practice further—help more people achieve better health *and* make more money—but they're stuck at a certain level.

Even the staff may not realize the shaky grounds upon which the practice rests, because the dentist hides these frustrations. But if something doesn't change, his fate will be to work until his final day—to die with drill in hand.

If this all sounds familiar, you might be asking yourself, *"How did I get here? And what am I supposed to do about it?"*

You probably prepared long and hard to gain entrance to dental school, endured years of schooling and perhaps a residency, until your education was complete.

And all that time you were going to school, you *weren't* making an income. By the time you were finally ready to hang out your shingle, you were heavily in debt and didn't own your own practice.

YOUR HIGH SCHOOL FRIEND, THE PLUMBER

Meanwhile, one high school friend became a plumber and commands $50 an hour. $50 per hour × 40 hours per week × 50 weeks per year × 6 years = $600,000

Assuming between undergrad and dental school, you accumulated $300,000-$400,000 in debt, and your plumber friend made $600,000, then there could be a million-dollar gap starting the day you graduate.

Dentistry can pay well, of course. Last year, the median annual wage for dentists was $158,120, according to the U.S. Bureau of Labor and Statistics.

But even if you make *twice* that—upwards of $300,000—you face a slew of expenses and unwelcome surprises.

Ever-increasing overhead, for one.

Plus, punishing PPO insurance rules, runarounds and reduced fees that can suck the profit (and the fun) out of your practice.

EVEN WHEN YOU'RE WITH YOUR FAMILY, ARE YOU REALLY THERE?

Maybe your spouse is losing patience because you're always at the office—or you're mentally there, even when you're with your family.

Is this message hitting home?

If so, this book can help you.

In the pages that follow, you're going to discover a whole new way of looking at these challenges. This clarity will transform your practice, and your life.

This book will reawaken hope that you can actually live your dreams by introducing you to special tools and super simple techniques I call "Gems."

Gems are easy, tactical practice management shortcuts. They don't take much of your time, but they do deliver massively outsized results—and lead you to the life you've been longing for.

IMAGINE WHAT THAT MIGHT MEAN FOR YOU...

Maybe it means pulling up to your brand-new vacation home (for which you paid cash) in a new Mercedes convertible...

Maybe it means proudly watching your daughter graduate from college, knowing that you managed to pay for her schooling out of cash flow and not leave her (or yourself) saddled with debt...

Or maybe it just means looking back on your career with warmth in your heart, because you improved the health and longevity of thousands of patients by providing exceptional dental care.

Whatever dream most inspires you, I want to take you one giant leap closer to making it a reality.

Here's what's ahead.

We'll begin with my story, because I was once in the situation that you're struggling with. (My darkest days may have been even worse than what you're facing now.)

Next, we'll take a look at the issues consuming your attention right now: issues like insurance company bullying, team member accountability, revenue and *profit* generation, and more.

Right here, right in this book, I'll give you keys to deal with those in the most efficient, effective and profitable way.

You'll also learn a new *conceptual framework*—this Gems idea we just discussed.

And I will give you *every* detail you'll need to immediately deploy a few amazingly simple Gems that will exponentially increase your revenue—and generate measurable increased revenue in *just a matter of days.*

Finally, we will explore the Gems mindset and survey additional ways to supercharge your practice. By the time we're done, you'll have a whole new toolbox at your disposal, and renewed hope and excitement for your future.

Let's dive in.

CHAPTER 1

FROM THE BRINK OF BANKRUPTCY TO BREAKTHROUGH

It was a cold, rainy, Friday afternoon 20 years ago. Things felt like they couldn't get any worse. If you've ever been there, you know it's one of the worst feelings ever. It's not your health, but it's just about everything else.

I was sitting across the desk from a Boston bankruptcy attorney. After evaluating my situation, he told me that declaring bankruptcy was the only way out of the financial and emotional dilemma I was in.

I was over $1,000,000.00 in debt. My wife had had enough and was demanding a divorce. She'd packed up our two small children and moved hours away.

Meanwhile, my office manager—the one team member who knew my dental practice was in real financial trouble—had embezzled what little money remained.

MY PERFECT STORM

As I look back at those days some 20 years ago... with overwhelming massive debt, embezzlement and divorce all happening at the same time, I often call that time in my life "My Perfect Storm."

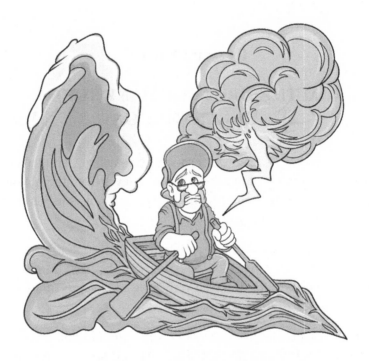

MY PERFECT STORM

"Meet me in court at 9 a.m. Monday," my attorney told me. But then, the next morning, I received a deeply troubling call from *another* lawyer—my divorce attorney.

FAILURE WAS NO LONGER AN OPTION

"Tom, you can't file for bankruptcy," he said. He'd been the one who referred me to the bankruptcy attorney, and he knew all about our meeting the day before.

"Your wife's lawyer just called," he explained. "He says if you do, he and your wife will go to family court and ask the judge to liquidate your home and dental practice."

"But that will leave me with nothing!" I said.

"I know," he said apologetically. "So, the risk of bankruptcy is just too great—you'll have to find another way out of your situation."

This seemed like the worst possible news at the time. Who would have thought I'd be *disappointed* that I couldn't go bankrupt?

And how had I gotten myself into this mess?

I had spent my first 15 years in practice focusing solely on perfecting my clinical skills. I admit that everything else—the business of dentistry, practice management, and especially the numbers—made my eyes glaze over.

Like many dentists I know, I figured that to grow the practice, I'd simply learn one more clinical technique, take another continuum, or buy some cool high-tech dental equipment. And that's what I did. I completed one continuum after another. But it didn't fix my problem; I kept sinking further into debt along the way.

Compounding the problem, I decided to take a deep dive into esthetic dentistry.

I devoted two years to preparing for the American Academy of Cosmetic Dentistry (AACD) accreditation exam. I became the first AACD-accredited dentist in Massachusetts. And I went on to serve as an AACD accreditation examiner for six years.

BECOMING CLINICALLY PROFICIENT DIDN'T PUT FOOD ON THE TABLE

I loved esthetic dentistry. But becoming the best clinical dentist I could be didn't put food on the table.

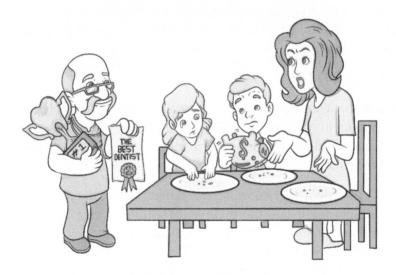

BEST DENTIST?

The hard truth is that I buried my head in the sand when it came to learning how to run a business, and because of that I spent every minute and dollar chasing my tail. So, when the bottom fell out of everything, my only recourse (I thought) was to declare bankruptcy.

When my attorney called to tell me my only remaining lifeline had been taken away, it felt like the end of the line.

But looking back today, his call was the best thing that ever happened to me.

With bankruptcy off the table, and two households to pay for (because of the divorce), I had to figure out another way.

I had to do something. Anything. But *what?*

I started exploring business "best practices." I went down rabbit hole after rabbit hole. But nothing seemed to apply particularly well to dentistry.

HOW A CLOGGED SINK LED ME TO DISCOVER A $100,000/YEAR GEM

Then one evening, my mom invited me over for dinner. I was grateful to hear about her world, and to focus on someone else's problems for a change. And to get a home cooked meal.

When I arrived, mom's kitchen sink was so clogged we had to call a plumber. I sat and waited while he did his thing, mildly agitated by the interruption.

As he finished up, my mother said, "Bill, while you're here, would you be willing to take a look at our toilet?"

He obliged. And then she added, "And while you're here, we've also got a drip in our shower. Can you help with that, too?"

He said sure, because my mom was charming, and hard to say no to. She kept hitting him with these "while you're here" requests.

By the time he left he'd taken care of several problems in addition to the clogged sink. He even gave her a new plunger as a thank you for all the work.

And this got me thinking.

14

My mother got rid of problems that had dogged her for months. The plumber got new, unexpected business, and a nice paycheck. And they both saved time, because they didn't have to schedule separate appointments.

Win-win.

THE "WHALYA" GEM IS BORN

"Whoa," I thought. "Could I do that in my practice somehow?"

"While you're here..." became shortened in my mind to WHALYA, because that's how my mom pronounced it—with the words slurred together. "WHALYA here..."

The next day I entered my office more energized than I'd been in months.

I called an impromptu staff meeting. "Do we have any time gaps today where we don't have patients back to back?" I asked. "Ten minutes here or there while I'm waiting for anesthetic to take, or impressions to set?"

"We'll have three or four spaces like that in today's schedule," my receptionist told me.

Great. It was GO time.

Our first "WHALYA" was a patient named Barbara. She'd come in for a cleaning. My hygienist noticed that she needed a small filling. Rather than schedule another appointment, she floated a WHALYA.

"Barbara, WHALYA here, want us to take care of that filling today so you won't have to make a separate trip?"

Barbara had three small kids at home, the sitter was already with them, and she appreciated that we were saving her an extra visit. With no hesitation she said, "Sure."

It was a simple moment—not a big deal at all. We squeezed in a few minutes to give a patient a filling she needed.

But it broke the dam.

We started instituting WHALYAs as a regular part of our day. We added one or sometimes two WHALYA patients every day. Six or seven patients per week... patients who otherwise would have been rescheduled to some day in the future.

Sometimes we'd work them into a small opening in the schedule. Other times I'd see them at strategic times alongside other patients.

HAPPIER PATIENTS AND A $100,000+ INCREASE IN REVENUE

At first, it was just a couple extra fillings here and there. An extraction. Once in a while there'd be a simple crown prep. It wasn't huge money each time—maybe $300 to $400 on average. But the *principle* excited me.

And it added up. In just a couple months, we were consistently generating $1,900 to $2,200 extra per week. That amounted to an *annual* jump of as much as *$110,000*!

More importantly, we were making our patients happier as a result.

Before this epiphany, I operated like most offices. When we finished with patients, we just took them out to the front desk and scheduled the next treatment for a future date. We didn't think twice about doing so.

It's what we were all taught to do. You perform your exam; you write up a plan; you take them out to the front desk; and you schedule.

But by ignoring this norm, I accrued $110,000 in *EXTRA* annual revenue.

I began wondering *what else might I be missing?*

I FELT LIKE I'D BEEN WORKING IN A COALMINE

Up until this point, running a dental practice felt like mining for coal, except all I was getting out was dirt and dust and exhaustion.

But with the WHALYAs, my perspective shifted. Working harder to extract more coal wasn't working, because *coal* wasn't the answer at all.

What I really needed were more things like WHALYAs. I needed to be mining for *Gems*. They're beautiful, they're worth more, and (I soon discovered) they're a lot less work.

But where could I find *more* Gems?

This question nagged at me.

At this point, I wasn't trying to turn the battleship. I still didn't have the heart or energy to do so. I just wanted to make small, quick, profitable changes based on *thinking differently.*

Shortly after implementing the WHALYA Gems in my practice, I attended a seminar by Dr. Gordon Christensen. Gordon offered fascinating clinical information, but I was daydreaming during his lecture. I needed more money. I needed to turn my practice around. His information was great but quite frankly it was hard for me to concentrate on what he was saying.

Then I heard something that struck me right between the eyes.

"Root caries..." he began.

"Root caries is like the beginning of the end of your tooth."

I knew that Fluoride delivered at the end of the prophy visit could help prevent the development of root caries.

I had been letting my patients down, as well as my practice. But because insurance doesn't cover Fluoride for adults, I had no idea how to convince patients they needed this treatment.

I KNEW ADULTS WOULD BENEFIT, BUT INSURANCE DIDN'T COVER

For weeks, I agonized.

I knew—or at least, I had a strong intuition—that if I could put together a compelling argument, I could convince some percentage of my patients to get Fluoride. But I wasn't sure what to say, how to say it, or whether this whole thing was even worth the time.

What kept me going was two things: necessity (I had to generate more revenue), and a desire to help people (I would never recommend a treatment that wouldn't profoundly improve the welfare of my patients).

I created a relatively weak first draft of my "Fluoride Verbal Skills," as I came to call them. I talked to my patients from the heart and explained the logic.

It was awkward at first, but several patients accepted the recommendation.

Soon, around 20% to 25% of my adults were paying for Fluoride out of pocket.

Okay, so I was onto something. How far could I take it?

I continued to wordsmith these Fluoride Verbal Skills, testing out variations, doing trial and error over three or four months. Finally, I arrived at an "optimized" process, which was routinely gaining an 80% (!) acceptance rate among patients.

And then I taught my hygienists to use this compelling language. And what do you know? It worked for them, too. Some achieved a nearly 100% acceptance rate with our patients.

7 SIMPLE SENTENCES ACHIEVE 80% ACCEPTANCE OF ADULT FLUORIDE PAID OUT-OF-POCKET

Eventually, I boiled the language down to just seven sentences: short enough to fit on a 3x5 card, clear enough that almost any hygienist could be trained to use it, and powerful enough that we would never again hear patients asking, "Does my insurance cover it?"

At the time, I had five hygienists between my two practices—three full-time and two part-time. With an 80% acceptance rate for Fluoride, we were doing a far better job of serving the health needs of our patients. *And* we started generating an increase of approximately $50,000 per (full-time) hygienist *per year*. Between my two offices, we added nearly $200,000 in revenue from adult Fluoride treatments per year—paid *out of pocket*.

I had found a way in. Finally. I had tasted success.

Not by digging for coal, but by looking at the world—at the dental profession—in new ways.

I came to realize that diamonds, rubies, emeralds, opals and sapphires were all around me. They're around all of us. Hiding in plain sight.

> *I want YOU to experience this same success.*
> *In a moment, right here in this book*
> *I will reveal, word for word, my*
> *Seven Simple Sentences Fluoride Verbal Skills.*
> *YOUR hygienist(s) can begin immediately helping*
> *your patients achieve better health, and,*
> *measurably increase your practice revenue.*

FORGET THE COALMINES. SCOOP UP THE GEMS.

By the end of that first year, I had picked up and carefully cut and polished five different Gems. And the impact was radical. My practice was saved. I had massive enthusiasm for the future for the first time in... I didn't know how long.

I had *made it*.

But my joy was cut short with a phone call.

My father had been taken to the hospital for what we thought was just a stomach ulcer. Diagnosis: terminal cancer.

My father wasn't a dentist, but he was the businessman owner of a dental practice about 45 minutes west of mine.

As I sat by his hospital bed, he took my hand and said, "Tom, I haven't been able to put anything away for your mother. Nothing. We have no retirement savings—I put it all into trying to save the practice. And it's now deeply in debt. I need you to promise me you'll take over and turn it around like you did your practice, so your mom will have something to live on."

My dad's practice—indeed, his entire approach to the profession—was radically different than mine. I had a small team, he had a huge staff. I had four operatories, he had 11 chairs. I was strictly fee-for-service, he'd signed with 15 PPOs and was 95% managed care. I was in a nice suburb of Boston, he was in an economically depressed urban environment.

Together with my new wife Elizabeth—whom I had met in the process of rebuilding—I headed out to his practice armed with Gems that had turned my practice around. But would they work in a practice so radically different than ours?

Indeed, they did. Within two years we were able to ramp up new patient flow, improve acceptance of best-option care, and eliminate 13 of his 15 PPOs.

Gems Family Members watch
GOLDMINE UNDERGROUND TEAM TRAINING TOOLKIT EPISODES 049 AND 050
"How to Triple New Patient Referrals"
AND EPISODE 053,
"Bobble Headed Dog Achieves Maximum Case Acceptance."

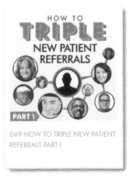

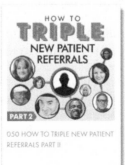

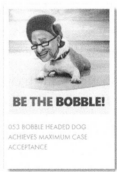

Most importantly, we were able to create a sound and secure financial future for my mom.

With my dad's practice back on track, another dentist friend of mine came to me and said, "I think it's amazing what you've done. Would you be willing to show me how to improve *my* practice?"

I said *sure*. And I did. And his practice took off, too.

All the while, I kept "Gem hunting"—searching for, collecting, and testing street level tactics for the practices.

And I realized this was my *true* calling.

If I experienced all this pain and uncertainty, as my dad and my friend had, then surely thousands of other dentists were going through it too.

What if I could help them increase the wealth and happiness they derived from their own practices, and in the process help their patients achieve optimal health as well? I could touch the lives of literally millions of people for the better.

And that's what's brought me to you.

DELIVER BETTER CARE, WORK LESS, AND MAKE MORE MONEY

I want *you* to benefit from these ideas. Because if they can help you and your team deliver better care *and* generate more revenue, have more fun and experience less stress, think what that will mean to you and your loved ones.

If you're under stress to make more money, if you want to work less and spend more time with your family or following your other passions, if you're tired of fighting with insurance companies... I am here to help.

More dentists than you can imagine face challenges identical to yours. And just like you, they've done everything they can to hide it from view.

The problems you face result from systemic issues that have nothing to do with your ability as a dentist, or how hard you've worked.

But don't fall into the trap of believing that those problems that seem so overwhelming require complex, expensive or unattainable solutions.

This was my next epiphany, and perhaps the most important. Little hinges swing big doors. And small Gems can bring huge rewards.

Simple, street-level guerrilla tactics—intelligently applied—are all you need to boost your financial position, reduce your hours, and begin living the life you've imagined.

Before you sign up for another continuing education continuum, or ponder getting an MBA, or even consider throwing in the towel altogether, discover how easy it is to have the practice you dream of. All it takes is a few simple Gems.

This book will show you exactly how and why to incorporate Gems into your practice.

My transformation has endured over the years. I've proven to myself that I can accomplish anything I choose. At age 61, I'm slightly *below* my high-school weight (6' 2" and currently 170 pounds). I play volleyball on two nationally ranked seniors' teams. I sold my practices at age 46, never having to work again unless I chose to. I achieved autonomy... and that's what I want for you. To be in a position financially to work only *if* you want, and only with *whom* you want.

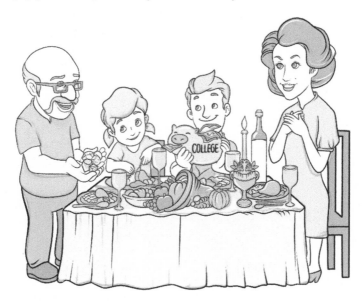

BEST PROVIDER

I have confidence in myself and my abilities as a father, a man, a provider—confidence I lacked prior to pushing through my Black Friday. I want you to experience the enduring sense of satisfaction and pride that I've been blessed to achieve.

The time to start is now...

CHAPTER 2

THE "GEMS PHILOSOPHY"

Do you remember studying the "simple machines" in school? You know—the pulley, the inclined plane, the wheel-and-axle?

The beauty of these mechanisms is that the force required when using them is less than the direct force would be to get something to move. A man might be unable to move a big rock or lift a heavy object all by himself. But if he has the right lever or pully, he can use just his own strength to move those things easily.

The same principle holds true in economics. Have you ever wondered why diamonds and emeralds and rubies are so valuable?

It's simple, really. Somewhere along the way, society developed a desire to possess these rare and beautiful items. They were coveted for the way they looked, and because they were hard to come by, they acquired great value. And that made them a symbol of wealth and status.

This meant that these gems were worth an immense amount in the marketplace and had a lot of trading power.

When civilization switched from the barter system to the idea of currency, gems could now be traded for lots of money— more than the cost and effort of finding and mining them. Gems acquired *leverage*. With a smaller amount of money or effort, they held a great deal of power.

This is the power of our Gems as well. They are actions requiring just a small amount of effort, but they have great value because they produce big results.

Remember in the previous chapter when I said I had been running my dental practice like I was mining for coal? Coal is useful, but it's not very valuable. You put in a lot of effort to dig it out, but it doesn't trade for very much. A handful of diamonds is worth more than several tons of coal, and labor-wise, it doesn't really take any more physical effort to mine a diamond than it does a piece of coal.

LEVERAGE YOUR TIME AND EFFORT, MAXIMIZE REVENUE

Most of us have been mining for coal in our practices, thinking, "That's just how it's done," not realizing that *we were standing in a field of Gems the whole time.*

Dentistry is more than just a practice. It's a *business.* Business-minded folks know that the best way to succeed in business isn't by grinding away at the same tasks day in and day out. It's by knowing how to leverage *maximum profits for minimal efforts.* It's the simple machine concept—a lot of results for a little bit of effort.

Here's the good news: There are Gems all around you—Gems you can use *right now* to increase your profits exponentially and turn your dental practice around. *You just have to know where to look for them.*

And here's MORE good news: You don't have to go on a treasure hunt to find them.

In the chapters that follow, I'm going to show you exactly where they are.

I'll start by handing you some of the easiest Gems you can use starting today. These alone can increase your revenue by *double or triple digits* within a year. In fact, if you put them to use right now, they'll start making money for you before you even finish this book.

So, let's get started with Gem #1: *WHALYAs*...

CHAPTER 3

WHALYAs

Once you begin looking, you'll realize there are constant opportunities to deploy one or more WHALYAs almost every day. It's simply a slight shift in your *mindset.*

Rather than *scheduling* a subsequent visit for each treatment you recommend, fit one or two of them into *today's* schedule. Your patients will be (far) happier and you will *easily* enjoy a $50,000.00 annual revenue increase with a potential $100,000.00 jump!

Once you've adopted the mindset, you'll have your team on the lookout for: a) places you can *fit* a WHALYA, and b) patients who might be happy to stay and get it done *now!*

Once you've determined who and when, the verbal skill is super simple. For example, at the end of the cleaning visit...

"Mary, WHALYA here, Dr. Smith could take care of that filling for you TODAY and save you a trip back."

"Bill, WHALYA here, if you like, Dr. Jones could take that tooth out and save you a trip."

"Susan, as long as you've already got your mom watching the baby, WHALYA here, Dr. Johnson could go ahead and start that crown for you today and save you a visit."

On the surface it seems simple enough. It's simple and effective *because* this Gem has been polished to perfection. In reality, it took nearly 18 months of trial and error to come up with the five words which we found had the most profoundly positive impact... *"Save you a trip back."*

Fact is, the *only* thing that matters to the patients is WIIFM... "What's in it for me?" What's the BIG BENEFIT to your patients? That said, I should point out that *if* you're dealing with a phobic patient, we found that adding another 9 words sealed-the-deal... *"And you won't lose one night's sleep over it!"*

"Mary, if you'd like to stay, Dr. Smith can take care of that for you right now and save you a trip back. And... you won't lose one night's sleep over it!"

WHALYAs ARE THE FIRST GEM

You'll find that many of your patients would *far* prefer to just get it done right then and there rather than have to come back. You eliminate the need to schedule an additional appointment (which they might not even keep), and you increase your revenue above what was planned for the day.

When you get in the habit of offering WHALYAs to your patients, you can easily add $1,000.00, possibly even $2000.00 revenue or more each week.

To be clear, WHALYAs are treatment you've: a) recommended to your patient anyway, b) they would otherwise have to come back for, and c) makes their life easier by doing it now instead of later.

A WHALYA is a true win-win. The patient appreciates the convenience of saving a trip and you generate more income... a far better use of your time, the one resource you can never replenish.

DR. KIRSTIN RAMSAY
AND THE "WHALYAs MINDSET"

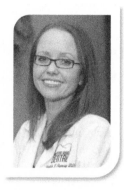

Before I met Tom, I struggled. I didn't have any systems in place. Training wasn't consistent. I was stressed out. Stuck. I couldn't figure out how to grow my practice.

I needed to make a change. I had the opportunity to hear Tom speak. His philosophy made sense to me. With Gems, choosing just a few little things, the *right* things, can make a really big difference. So, I jumped in.

Tom's concepts are very clear, which made his ideas easy to communicate. We began to speak with one voice... yet we didn't sound like machines. Our personalities still shined through. Once my team began to see the results from Gems, momentum built quickly.

Tom's "WHALYAs Challenge" kept WHALYAs top of mind for everybody, every day. We kept on the lookout for WHALYA opportunities, all the time.

Tom's unique approach helps us to use best practices. Now we're truly giving our patients the care they need, and, at a time that's more convenient for *them* (now versus rescheduling). A win-win... since performing treatment as WHALYAs (instead of scheduling another visit) has been *far* more profitable for our practice.

Each day, we ask ourselves, *"How can we optimize patient treatments?" And how can we serve our patients best?"* WHALYAs—and Gems in general—are a mindset. Tom provides us new and different ways to think, and to continue to grow our practice and our revenue.

—DR. KIRSTIN RAMSAY, Frisco, Texas

P.S. In addition to the increase we've enjoyed from WHALYAs, thanks to Tom's Fluoride Verbal Skills, 85% of my adult patients— sometimes even 90%—accept and pay for Fluoride regularly.

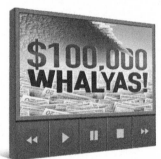

**THIS PRACTICE TRANSFORMING ACTION STEP WILL
VIRTUALLY GUARANTEE HAPPIER PATIENTS,
WHILE ADDING A POTENTIAL
$100,000 ANNUAL WINDFALL!**

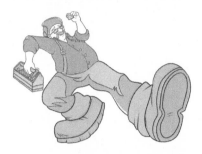

STOP READING. IT'S TIME TO TAKE ACTION!

Reading this book might be entertaining but won't make much of a difference in your life *unless* you STOP AND TAKE ACTION!

1. **Watch the WHALYAs VIDEO TEAM TRAINING** with your entire team. www.GemsAreEasy.com/VIDEOS

2. **Meet with your team to IDENTIFY WHEN and WHAT.**
    WHALYAs are a business *system*. In fact, one of *the* easiest most profitable systems you will ever deploy. As dentists, all we have to sell is our time. At the end of the day, time unused is lost forever.

    Meet with your team this afternoon. Look at tomorrow's schedule. Where in the schedule could you fit in a simple filling, an easy extraction, possibly even an initial crown prep? Once they know the what and where, it's just a matter of *who!* Now instead of ending Mrs. Jones' recall visit with, "Let's schedule that filling for you as soon as possible..." your team can say, "Mrs. Jones, WHALYA here, would you like to SAVE A TRIP and take care of that right now?"

3. **TRACK WHALYAs ADDED each week.** It's not at all unusual for Gems Family members to add one simple WHALYA each day. $400 x 5 days = $2,000 x 50 weeks = $100,000 each and every year!

CHAPTER 4

FLUORIDE VERBAL SKILLS

I'm just going to come out and say it. Insurance companies are way behind (or simply don't care about) the research when it comes to Fluoride treatments.

We've known for decades that Fluoride is critical to the development of children's teeth, especially between the ages of 6 months and 16 years. Fluoride helps build and restore a strong mineral layer in the tooth enamel, making incoming adult teeth more resistant to cavities.

But more recent research has also shown that Fluoride treatments are extremely beneficial for adults as well. Although our adult teeth aren't developing anymore, they are still susceptible to mineral erosion and cavities, especially root caries. Fluoride treatments administered immediately after a cleaning can help to prevent root caries, helping adult patients avoid lots of dental problems. In fact, since we are adults for a lot longer than we are children, it could even be argued that Fluoride treatments are *just as critical for adults as they are for children*—perhaps even more so.

So... why don't more of us recommend Fluoride treatments to our adult patients? Simple: *Insurance companies won't pay for it.*

We have allowed our dental practices to become so dependent on our patients' insurance that if a service isn't covered, we become skittish about offering it.

DOES MY INSURANCE COVER IT?

Many of us have tried to offer Fluoride treatments to our adult patients. But inevitably the question arises:

"Does my insurance cover it?"

"Unfortunately, not," we reply.

"Then no, thank you."

After a time, most of us get tired of hitting our heads against that wall, and we simply stop asking. I have to admit, I was just as guilty as anyone else. For years, I just never brought up the subject of Fluoride because I assumed the answer would be no.

It was only after my epiphany that I realized what a mistake I was making. *Not only was I denying my patients a very valuable treatment by default; over the years I was leaving hundreds of thousands of dollars on the table in the process.* That was money I definitely could have used when my practice was on the verge of closing.

Insurance isn't the real problem here. The fact is, our adult patients *need* Fluoride treatments, and most can afford to pay for them out-of-pocket. *The problem is that we haven't known how to present it.*

And that's the second Gem I want to put in your hand. I want to share exactly how to offer Fluoride treatments to your adult patients in a way that will *convince as many as 80 percent of them to say yes.*

SEVEN SIMPLE SENTENCES

When I first began offering Fluoride to my adult patients again, figuring out how to word the offer was really a trial-and-error process. I repeatedly tweaked and re-tweaked my approach until I found the right way to educate my patients on why they needed the treatment.

As I made adjustments, I started seeing better and better results—a few yesses here and there, then 20% acceptance, then 30%. Eventually, the pitch evolved into just *Seven Simple Sentences* that our team easily committed to memory.

Today, thousands of hygienists in the USA and around the world use my Seven Simple Sentences to routinely achieve *80 percent (or better) acceptance* of their recommendations of Fluoride from their adult patients.

Yes, you read that right. Eighty percent of dental patients say yes to Fluoride after teeth cleanings—and they all gladly pay out of pocket. Insurance be damned. It's that easy.

What does it mean in terms of dollars and cents? Our offices have seen average increase in revenue of *$50,000 per year, per hygienist*. We had the equivalent of four hygienists operating out of my two offices—for an extra $200,000 per year, for a few minutes of extra effort per patient.

I'm going to save you all the trial-and-error I went through crafting these Seven Simple Sentences. Just for reading this book, my **Fluoride Verbal Skills are my GIFT TO YOU** so you can start using them in your practice right away.

I've reprinted the *exact verbal skills* for you to share with your hygienists in order to achieve an instant improvement in your patients' health—and to make a lot more money. It takes the average hygienist just 30 minutes to learn these Seven Simple Sentences by heart. In order to easily commit them to memory *and* have all team members on the same page, we recommend practicing them out loud, round robin, with the entire team.

When your hygienists deploy these skills, most of your adult patients will soon be enthusiastically accepting—and paying out of pocket—for Fluoride treatments.

Here are The Seven Simple Sentences:

FLUORIDE VERBAL SKILLS

Mrs. Jones, recent research has helped us to uncover one of THE most devastating adult dental problems. The problem is known as **ROOT CAVITIES.** All adults are susceptible to root cavities.

One of the most respected dental researchers in the world says that once you get a cavity on your root surface, it's like the **BEGINNING OF THE END OF YOUR TOOTH.** Sure, we'll try to fix it, but even after we think we've removed all the cavity or decay, it often creeps up again right under the filling or crown… and we have to cut it out further and further up under the gum near the bone.

Problem is, **YOUR ROOTS ARE 1000% SOFTER THAN YOUR ENAMEL.** As an adult, you tend to have some recession of the gums…. That's when your gum drifts higher up the tooth and exposes some of your root… often early recession is so small it's not immediately apparent… **RECESSION DOESN'T HAVE TO BE VISIBLE** to put your tooth at risk!

The **BEST PREVENTION FOR ROOT CAVITIES IS FLUORIDE**… and the best and **MOST RELIABLE FLUORIDE DELIVERY IS IMMEDIATELY** after your cleaning… due to a natural film layer the body coats your teeth with, within 24 hours after your cleaning… the best time for Fluoride is at the end of your cleaning. This sticky substance decreases the ability of the Fluoride to penetrate into, and protect your teeth.

In fact, Mrs. Jones, we recently had a patient (first name), only 40 years old, who LOST a tooth due to this disease. Fact is that **WE HAD EFFECTIVE FLUORIDE FOR MANY YEARS**… BUT… they were SO incredibly acid **BITTER TASTING** that most adults refused to use them… myself included! **THE OLD FLUORIDE** took from 5 to 7 minutes in your mouth, and it was pretty close to **INTOLERABLE.**

We are fortunate today, to have **FAST ACTING HIGH STRENGTH** Fluorides that are extremely effective, but **TASTE GREAT** and require only **60 SECONDS.** I wouldn't allow my family or myself ever again to have a cleaning, without **IMMEDIATELY** afterwards having the Fluoride as well.

Insurance doesn't cover Fluoride for adults… but it's like having your OWN insurance policy to help insure keeping your natural teeth for life. The charge is $XX (do not pause here!) WE have mint, bubblegum, and raspberry, and strawberry… **WHICH DO YOU PREFER?**

GemsAreEasy.com/Book5

Dr. Tom "The Gems Guy" Orent

These Seven Simple Sentences have helped tens of thousands of patients attain better dental health and have generated millions of dollars of revenue for the dentists who use them. They're yours now, to use in good faith.

By mastering this Gem and using it in your practice, you'll be providing better care for your patients, reducing and preventing root caries, and you'll easily experience an increase of $40,000 to $50,000 per hygienist in annual revenue.

ADULT FLUORIDE AND TEAM BONUS – JUST 2 OF THE GEMS THAT HELPED PROPEL DR. STEPHEN JARVIE'S REVENUE BY 45%!

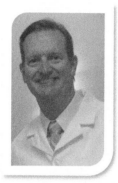

I've been practicing for about 27 years. What began as a feeling of malaise turned into desperation around the end of 2017.

I wasn't producing enough. I was disorganized, I didn't have good direction, and my leadership wasn't there. I was working 65 or 70 hours a week. I didn't have much of a home life. I wasn't happy and was in jeopardy of losing my practice.

I had worked with many coaches before this, and I'd read a lot of books. They all meant well, but they couldn't move my practice.

Then I found Tom. He helped us rapidly ramp up our production while ensuring that we gave our patients better treatment. I saw a big difference within the first month or two. And then it *really* took off...

The first Gem I used was so easy! **Adult Fluoride Verbal Skills**. It really worked, and my crew ran with it. Tom's team was very helpful. We had our own personal concierge. Whenever we had a question, our Concierge responded right away by emails or phone.

Tom's Team Bonus System and the Gems program in general have empowered the whole practice. Everybody, from the front desk to the patients, feels like they're part of something that really matters. That we make a difference in people's lives.

The staff started to enjoy their work; people were more positive in the office; and this enthusiasm translated into more productivity.

In the final quarter last year, we were up 45% from the previous year!

Tom shares great Gems on everything from verbal skills to leadership and psychology. I've grown as a leader and feel far more respected in the office than just a year ago.

I went into a lot of debt when I built my solo practice. There were times where I didn't feel like coming to work at all. But thanks to the transformation that resulted from working with Tom and implementing his Gems, I _love_ coming to work now.

My team loves the process as well. They are having more fun, laughing more. Being a part of the Gems Family has really bonded us more as an office. A team.

I plan to continue with Gems for a long time, because it's been so helpful. I feel like Tom and his team are part of our practice. I really do.

—_DR. STEPHEN J. JARVIE, Novi, Michigan_

You could be getting results just like Dr. Jarvie, with no risk, cost or obligation. For details go to:

www.GemsAreEasy.com/Book5

THIS PRACTICE TRANSFORMING ACTION STEP WILL HELP YOUR PATIENTS ACHIEVE BETTER HEALTH AND COULD ADD $50,000 ANNUAL REVENUE!

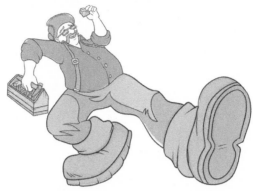

STOP READING. IT'S TIME TO TAKE ACTION!

Reading this book might be entertaining but won't make much of a difference in your life *unless* you STOP AND TAKE ACTION!

1. **Photocopy the seven simple sentence Fluoride Verbal Skills** from this chapter. Hand one copy to each of your team members (*not* just the hygienist!).

2. **Watch the Fluoride Verbal Skills VIDEO TEAM TRAINING** with your entire team. **www.GemsAreEasy.com/VIDEOS**

3. **Invest just 15 to 20 minutes in VERBAL SKILLS TRAINING.** Meet with your team and have *each* member "role play" the Fluoride Verbal Skills to another team member acting as the patient.

4. **Have your RDH(s) DEPLOY the Fluoride Verbal Skills** with your adult patients during prophy visits.

5. **TRACK acceptance each week.** How many accepted divided by how many were offered = acceptance. Within just a few weeks you should achieve roughly 80% acceptance!

CHAPTER 5

PUTTING THE GEMS TO WORK IN YOUR PRACTICE

I hope you're beginning to understand the true power of Gems, and how they can revolutionize the success of your dental practice. If you stop reading this book right now and implement just the two Gems I've shared with you thus far—WHALYAs and Fluoride Verbal Skills—you can easily increase your annual revenue by a *minimum* of $100,000, and possibly $200,000 or more.

But that's just the start. There are many more Gems you can put to use. Each one has the potential on its own to dramatically increase your bottom line. At the same time, these Gems are all highly beneficial to your patients' oral health. By using them, you'll be building a community of loyal, happy patients who not only come back to you again and again, but who will gladly recommend you and your practice to their friends and family.

I've discovered and developed hundreds of practice-growing Gems. Here are just a sampling of some of them...

The Periodontal Verbal Skills GEM

GOLDMINE UNDERGROUND TEAM TRAINING TOOLKIT EPISODE 052

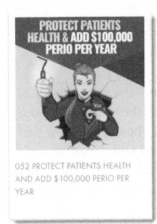

052 PROTECT PATIENTS HEALTH AND ADD $100,000 PERIO PER YEAR

Most general dental practices grossly underserve the periodontal needs of their patients.

These patients suffer the ravages of gum disease, damage to underlying bone, and potential loss of teeth. Gum disease, even in its early stages, causes low level bacteremia (blood-borne infection), which can double the risk of heart attack and stroke, increase the risk of early onset Alzheimer's, and wreak havoc with blood sugar control and diabetes.

EDUCATING PATIENTS REGARDING THE ORAL-SYSTEMIC LINK

Our understanding of the oral systemic link has become one of the most important breakthroughs of modern dentistry. Gum disease contributes to a long list of health issues, some of which can be fatal.

As dental practitioners, it is our role—and our moral obligation—to stem this tide of negative health consequences associated with periodontal infection.

How do we do that?

We communicate with patients empathetically, effectively, and systematically, so they care for themselves and make healthier choices. To that end:

- Every adult patient should have a complete periodontal probing and charting as a component of every hygiene visit.

- Communicate *your* periodontal protocol with your team. In each practice, doctors must set a "periodontal decision line protocol"—the level of pocketing, bleeding etc., a minimum bar above which the hygienist should begin the discussion about the need for Perio Phase I treatment.

  Of course, the doctor will still make the final diagnosis... but <u>patients are *far* more accepting of the need for care in the absence of symptoms when that need is first raised by the *hygienist*</u> as opposed to the doctor.

- We need to influence our patients, clearly and ethically, to accept our recommendations for their continued health and wellbeing.

Including this process as part of your overall hygiene program will help your patients *and* generate a new flow of revenue.

Let's say your hygienist performs Perio Phase I treatments on **just two additional patients per week**. Ensuring the health and longevity of those patients can translate into approximately **$100,000.00 increased revenue** per year.

Not bad.

I've designed a simple, step-by-step method of achieving these results by deploying my Periodontal Verbal Skills (and graphics) Team Training Toolkit. If you'd like to give this powerful Gem a try and see the results for yourself, just go to www.GemsAreEasy.com/Book5 and take a FREE 6-Week Test Drive of my Gems Platinum Team Training Toolkit.

A TEAM BONUS SYSTEM THAT WORKS!

In his bestselling book *Good to Great*, Jim Collins observed that the most successful businesses—including dental and professional practices—have a big thing in common. *They build and value great teams.*

According to Collins' analysis, having the right people doing the right things is even more valuable than having a compelling vision. Without great people, you cannot build an enduring institution.

But great people are hard to find. It's not an accident that the top CEOs of the top companies in the world spend up to 30% or 40% of their time recruiting.

One of the best ways to recruit and keep and delight a team is to implement an appropriate bonus system.

You can't expect your best employees to learn and deploy new skills—and to help your practice grow and thrive—without any chance of enjoying the rewards of your success. You need to include your personnel in the rewards their work has generated.

A strong bonus system also encourages employees to spread the word about your practice to their network. That makes it easier to recruit great people, and to acquire even more patients.

The Team Bonus System Gem does this for you—often just by simply making a small, tactical tweak to your practice.

Expecting your team to help you maximize the enormous opportunities in your practice in the absence of a proven-effective Team Bonus System is like expecting water to magically appear *before* you've primed the pump.

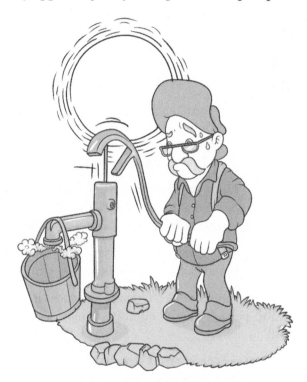

NOTHING BUT DUST

Making these slight adjustments (like the Team Bonus System) can energize your personnel in the same way a magnifying glass tilted at the right angle to the sun can start a fire.

That's exactly what happened to Dr. Scott when she began implementing just this one powerful Gem...

Dr. Alison Scott's Quest
For a Team Bonus System that Works

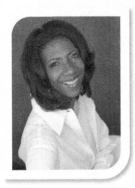

I felt like the hamster in the cage, just spinning my wheels. I have an associate who's been with me through thick and thin—but I was still missing a big piece of the practice success puzzle.

Then I had the good fortune of finding Tom Orent. I saw the amazing results other doctors were getting with his program and I knew I had to try his Gems.

Tom's wife Elizabeth got me excited about Gems' Team Bonus System 2.0. This was dearly needed. And my team members were really *excited* when I told them about it.

I had struggled forever trying to create an effective employee incentive structure. I tried *many* different bonus systems.

It was Gems' Team Bonus System 2.0 that finally nailed it. The team looks forward to payroll. There's an attitude now of, "Great, it's Monday again!"

The beauty of the Gems approach is that it's like a smorgasbord of brilliant techniques and strategies to choose from. You can always find the Gems that are the best fit for *your* practice.

I'm excited about the future of the practice. I'm on track. I really enjoy being a part of the Gems Family, the help they offer, and the retreats where we get together. We just learn so much!

I didn't realize just how well we were doing until recently when I dove into the numbers. When I compared our revenue to what we had done the year before, I was like, "Wow, I can't believe this!"

—DR. ALISON SCOTT, Houston, Texas

1-888-880-GEMS (4367)

Want to stop feeling like a "hamster in a cage" like Dr. Scott? It's easier than you think!

Go to www.GemsAreEasy.com/Book5 for details about a game changing FREE offer.

Of course, you can experiment with different compensation structures, and maybe you'll discover a bonus system of your own that will empower and motivate your team.

How to Get My Team Bonus System FREE

GOLDMINE UNDERGROUND TEAM TRAINING TOOLKIT EPISODE 046

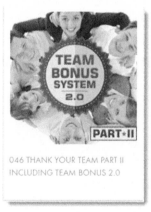

046 THANK YOUR TEAM PART II
INCLUDING TEAM BONUS 2.0

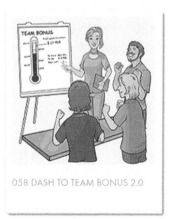

058 DASH TO TEAM BONUS 2.0

If you want to bypass the time (and lost revenue) these experiments entail, and instead move immediately to success, a **FREE 6-WEEK TEST DRIVE** of Gems Family Platinum can help you. Go to www.GemsAreEasy.com/Book5

During your FREE Test Drive of Gems Platinum, we'll show you exactly how to establish a Team Bonus System and make it work for your practice.

We'll not only show you how it works, we'll *create* your Team Bonus System Calculator... Done-For-You. My wife,

Elizabeth, "The Engineer" and your Personal Gems concierge
will show you exactly how to use it.

All you'll need to do is drop your team's numbers for the week
into your Bonus System Calculator and the rest is automatic.
We've calibrated this through real world testing in hundreds
of dental practices across the country, to constantly monitor
and improve its effectiveness.

I've mentioned the "Free Test Drive." But far more important
to me is that you **understand conceptually** what these
Gems are and why they work.

As you'll see, Gems are all very simple. They're easy to
understand, fast to implement and not at all disruptive. They
are all designed to improve your patients' health *and* to
generate revenue rapidly and consistently. Both the Fluoride
Verbal Skills and the Periodontal Verbal Skills have proven
effective over the past two decades, in thousands of practices,
in 48 countries.

When you unite these with the Team Bonus System Gem that
compensates your team smartly, so that they win when your
patients opt for better care, **magic** happens.

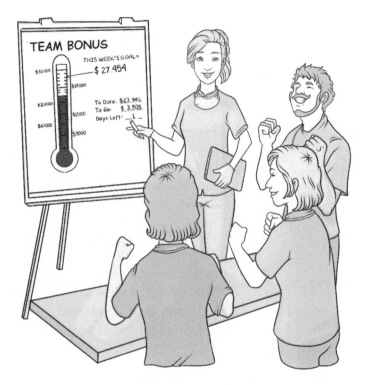

RALLYING THE TEAM

How to Double Hygiene Recall

GOLDMINE UNDERGROUND TEAM TRAINING TOOLKIT EPISODE 009

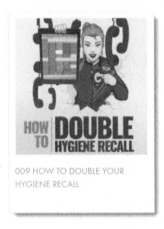

009 HOW TO DOUBLE YOUR HYGIENE RECALL

Hygiene recall is the engine that drives the most successful dental practices. Show me a tremendously successful dental office and 99% of the time, I'll show you a practice with a thriving hygiene department.

Our team has done in-depth analyses of thousands of dental practices over the past 20 years. The evidence clearly shows that when hygiene is thriving, the cash flow increases, and the resulting diagnosed, scheduled and treated restorative is exponentially greater.

My team training toolkit, "How to Double Hygiene Recall," can rapidly boost this core piece of your practice. It's not unusual for my Gems Family Members to add 10 or even 15 hours of jam-packed hygiene visits into their weekly schedules. That's an extra day or two per week.

This can mean a shot in the arm of $150,000 or $200,000 in annual revenue. Those figures take into account about $75,000 in RDH production and another $125,000 or so in doctor production from the restorative treatment produced by all those extra recall exams.

The training about recall consists of two Gems—two small tweaks—that I teach dentists to make. Let's walk through them, and then we'll wrap up this piece of the book.

TAILORING HYGIENE RECALL FREQUENCY BASED ON INDIVIDUAL PATIENTS' HEALTH NEEDS

Most practices have the majority of their patients on a 6-month recall schedule. Ask dentists or dental team members, and most will tell you they just assumed a 6-month recall rate was designed by the dental insurance industry. Nope!

This 6-month interval was arbitrarily conceived by a guy working in the Pepsodent marketing department—back in the 1930s! He came up with a tag line: *"See your dentist twice a year, and brush with Pepsodent twice a day."* Before that there was no protocol for "regular" visits to the dentist.

Many dental insurance companies—in fact, most—have astonishingly adopted Pepsodent's two-times-a-year cleaning as their standard for reimbursement. Think about that. An 80+ year-old toothpaste commercial defines the gold standard of dental recall care in America. Insane.

Here's why this is so bad.

As you probably know, many adults would benefit *greatly* from more frequent cleanings. Some people should visit *minimally* every three months. For instance:

- Diabetics
- Those who have a family or personal history of heart disease or stroke
- Those who've had a transient ischemic attack (TIA)
- Those with a family history of Alzheimer's

We offer a Special Report on the Oral-Systemic Link, titled "29 Classifications of Your Patients that MUST Be on 3-Month Recall."

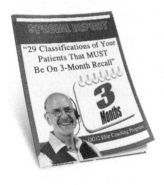

You get instant access to this report with your **FREE 6-Week Test Drive** of my Gems Platinum Team Training Toolkit. Go to: www.GemsAreEasy.com/Book5

But knowing who these patients *are* is just the first step. You also must develop specific, motivating language to convey to these patients *why* they must come back more often than every six months.

And the verbal skills are slightly different for each classification of patient. For some it's just a matter of improved oral health. For others, it can be the difference between life and death.

In the "29 Classifications" report you'll find easy to use proven effective verbal skills with which to help your patients understand why they'll benefit from more frequent recall... based upon *their* specific situation as it relates to the oral-systemic link.

These Recall Verbal Skills are similar to the Fluoride Verbal Skills. During your FREE Test Drive as a Gems Family Platinum Member, you'll have access to my team Training Toolkit, "How to Double Hygiene Recall," which includes my step-by-step training on exactly how to do this.

You'll also receive the "29 Classifications" special report, so that you and your team can deploy the skills to the right patients with pinpoint precision.

The second strategy for increasing recalls isn't analyzed in depth here, but is thoroughly detailed in my Team Training Toolkit, "How to Double Hygiene Recall."

If your practice is sending out postcards, letters, emails or text reminders of recall appointments, keep at it. But there is a simple change to your recall system that will generate from eight to fifteen or more recall patients each week by creating a paradigm shift in the way you make **hygiene recall phone calls**.

This is also included when you sign up for your **6-WEEK FREE TEST DRIVE** of Gems Family Platinum Membership at www.GemsAreEasy.com/Book5

GEMS THEORY OF "THE BOBBLE-HEADED DOG"

I'm sure you've been stopped at a traffic light and seen one of those little bobble-headed dogs on the rear windshield deck of the car in front of you?

Earlier, when discussing Perio Phase I protocol, I mentioned that patients are *far* more accepting of the need for care in the absence of symptoms when that need is first raised by the hygienist.

This concept is *not* limited to the diagnosis of periodontal disease (which in its early to moderate stages is *often* asymptomatic). It applies to the *vast* majority of dental problems. As general dentists, 95% of the care we render is aimed at solving problems for which there are *no* symptoms.

For example: wide open leaking margins on a 25-year-old failed-in-place amalgam; incipient caries diagnosed using Diagnodent, SOPROLIFE, Canary, or CariVu; deep dentin fracture diagnosed using transillumination... most if not *all* of these common problems present without symptoms. It's not at all uncommon to hear a new patient say, "Doc, I'm pretty sure everything's just fine... think all I need is a cleaning and a quick checkup!"

Translation... the patient has no clue she has periodontal disease, recurrent caries on three teeth and a deep dentin fracture on an old MODBL amalgam... time bomb just waiting to explode!

WHY MANY PATIENTS SILENTLY ASSUME WE MAY BE RECOMMENDING WORK WHERE NONE MAY BE NEEDED

When performing a prophy and exam on an *asymptomatic* patient... if the hygienist completes the prophy and never mentions word one about any of the above issues and then you walk in the room and tell the patient she needs $3,000.00 worth of treatment... guess what the patient is thinking (and sometimes even says out loud)?

"Doc, you need a new BMW?"

"Hey doc, are you building a new home?"

"What? You want me to pay your son's tuition to Harvard?"

Fact is, no matter how wonderful the doctor-patient relationships we build, many asymptomatic patients' first reaction is that we are finding work to do in order to make more money.

With respect to most of the routine issues we see every day, when your hygienist is well-trained with effective verbal skills appropriate for each diagnosis and potential treatment, you and I (doctors) become just a second opinion when we enter the room!

Patients "pre-heated" by the hygienist are far more accepting of doctors' recommendations when we simply walk into the room and, shaking our heads up and down... agree with our hygienists' findings and recommendations (thus "The Bobble-Headed Dog!").

We were *never* taught to do this in dental school. In fact, NONE of the business building Gems I share with my thousands of Gems Family Member dentists were taught to us in dental school!

But I can assure you from my own dental practices and the experience of thousands of Gems Family Member dentists who've deployed this Gem, you *will* experience higher case acceptance when patients no longer see you as just out to make more money. In their eyes you will become what we know in our hearts you already were... a "TRUSTED ADVISOR."

HYGIENISTS CANNOT LEGALLY DIAGNOSE OR TREATMENT PLAN

But wait! Tom, it's not legal in my state for a hygienist to diagnose or treatment plan. Got it. Actually, it's not legal in *any* of the 50 United States (and likely nowhere in the world). I'm not an attorney, so check with yours if you wish, but here's what I taught my five hygienists to say immediately before telling a patient what they saw and may recommend...

"Mary, I'm not a dentist so I can't diagnose or treatment plan, however I've been working with Dr. Orent for seven years and I've seen this (perio, open margins, deep dentin fracture, etc.) a thousand times, and I can tell you what he's going to say when he walks into the room..."

At which point they inform the patient about the problems they see and the most likely solutions I'll be recommending when I come in for the exam. Again, we're not talking about having hygienists attempt to treatment plan complex full-mouth care, perio-prosth, etc. this is your routine bread and butter, Phase I perio, build-ups and crowns, fillings, etc.

FREE TEAM TRAINING VIDEO
BOBBLE-HEADED DOG ACHIEVES
MAXIMUM CASE ACCEPTANCE!
GOLDMINE UNDERGROUND TEAM TRAINING TOOLKIT EPISODE 053

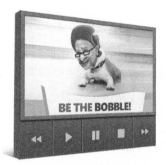

As general dentists, 95% of the problems we diagnose and the treatment we recommend is found in the *absence* of symptoms.

No doubt you have an amazing relationship with your patients. But when it comes to opening their wallets for care you recommend to an asymptomatic patient, YOUR PATIENTS WILL TRUST YOUR HYGIENIST MORE than they trust you.

Allow me to train your team *for* you on my "Theory of the Bobble-Headed Dog." When your hygienist is the *first* to mention the need for care in the absence of symptoms, then you enter the room as a second opinion simply *confirming* what she has already stated, YOUR CASE ACCEPTANCE AND PRACTICE REVENUE WILL INCREASE!

Be my guest and watch the same step-by-step detailed VIDEO TEAM TRAINING TOOLKIT my Gems Family members enjoy. After watching this video your team will understand *why* it's critical they lay out the groundwork for the need for care in the absence of symptoms *before* you enter the room. I'll train your hygienist with quick, simple verbal skills. Watch your case acceptance skyrocket!

To watch the FREE VIDEO, go to **www.GemsAreEasy.com/VIDEOS**

THIS PRACTICE TRANSFORMING ACTION STEP WILL MEASURABLY IMPROVE CASE ACCEPTANCE AND HELP YOUR PATIENTS ACHIEVE BETTER HEALTH!

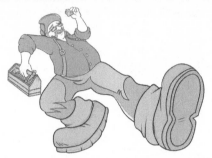

STOP READING. IT'S TIME TO TAKE ACTION!

Reading this book might be entertaining but won't make much of a difference in your life *unless* you STOP AND TAKE ACTION!

1. **Watch the Bobble-Headed Dog VIDEO TEAM TRAINING** with your entire team. **www.GemsAreEasy.com/VIDEOS**

2. **Invest just 15 to 20 minutes in your RDH(s) re: Deployment**.

   a. Train the initial verbal skill, "Mary, I'm not a dentist so I can't diagnose or treatment plan, but I've been working with..."

   b. Review the *basic* most common problems and the treatments you routinely plan when encountered so you and your hygienists are on the same page

3. **Have your RDH(s) DEPLOY the Bobble-Headed Dog protocol.** You'll be amazed at your patients' positive reaction to hearing about these issues *first* from your hygienist and *then* from you.

4. **TRACK acceptance each week.** How many patients scheduled treatment divided by how many were offered = case acceptance. Watch your case acceptance *measurably* improve!

How to Eliminate the Stress of the Hygiene Recall Exam

GOLDMINE UNDERGROUND TEAM TRAINING TOOLKIT EPISODE 055

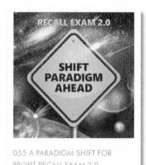

055 A PARADIGM SHIFT FOR PROFIT RECALL EXAM 2.0

Back in my first clinical year of dental school, we were learning how to perform a prophy. The instructors would come in at the end of the visit to see if we'd removed all the calculus. Since the dawn of time, dentists have been following this same model to check their hygienists' work with patients.

Working with dentists and team members for more than 20 years, I've heard the following complaints over and over: *doctors* complain that their hygienists don't consistently complete all the steps they should during hygiene recall visits; and *hygienists* complain that the doctors are asking them to do more tasks than they can possibly complete... *and* doctors mess up hygienists' schedules by keeping them waiting when it's time for the recall exam.

The solution is quite simple. Here are the 3 steps:

1. **SCHEDULE A FULL HOUR**

   Ensure that adults are scheduled for a full hour for recall examination and prophy. You're probably already doing this.

   But occasionally I've come across doctors who figured they'd save and make more money if they only allowed

45 or 50 minutes for recall. This is a *false sense of savings.*

There are *dozens* of other "false sense of savings" mistakes dentists are making that are costing them hundreds of thousands of dollars per year. To discover the errors you are making and how to easily eliminate them go to www.GemsAreEasy.com/Book5 for a **FREE 6-Week Test Drive** of my Gems Platinum Team Training Toolkit.

When you give your hygienist sufficient time to complete the examination steps and prophy, you'll increase the amount of restorative dentistry being put back into the doctor's chair.

2. **HYGIENIST: BEGIN WITH THE EXAMINATION!**

Have your hygienist begin the recall visit by completing every examination step (radiographs, photos, perio probing, etc.) that you require. That should take 15 minutes at most.

Then your hygienist alerts you that she's ready for you to join her for the reexam. You now have a huge 45-minute window within which you can get in to do the exam.

You don't need to check whether your hygienist removed the calculus adequately. The fact is, our hygienists do a far better job cleaning teeth than we ever would.

And it won't take you nearly as long to perform that exam when your hygienist has already laid the groundwork for patient acceptance, using the appropriately scripted verbal skills and graphics before you walk in the room (my "Theory of the Bobble-Headed Dog").

3. **DON'T CONFUSE PROPHY WITH PERIODONTAL TX**

   The 2nd leading cause of dental malpractice lawsuits is a dentist's failure to diagnose and treat periodontal disease. What is a *prophy* supposed to be anyway? It's a supragingival scaling and polishing of the crowns of the teeth in a healthy periodontia.

   If your patient has significant subgingival calculus, pocketing, and bleeding, it means they have a periodontal infection, which should be treated as such with multiple visits under anesthetic! Otherwise the procedure will hurt, and not do them nearly the therapeutic good that they need.

The Gems we've gone over are just the tip of the iceberg. These are not theoretical tools. They are battle-tested, easy to deploy, simple changes that you can make now.

You don't have to take a month-long CE course to learn a new technique or advanced technology. Gems are *simple* fixes. So simple they may almost seem trivial. But there is magic in simplicity, when it's the *right* simplicity.

How hard is it to memorize seven sentences on a 3 x 5 index card? Or to watch a short video with your team?

THE ANSWER: GEMS ARE EASY!

If you haven't started, go out now and test the Fluoride Verbal Skills or the WHALYA Gems. That's all you need to begin generating revenue.

And if you'd like more of my help building your practice, and achieving the *life* of your dreams, I invite you to take the free test drive to access the other Gems discussed in this chapter (and much more). Go to www.GemsAreEasy.com/Book5

THE BLACK HOLE OF NO-SHOWS & LAST-MINUTE CANCELLATIONS

Think about what happens when **one of your patients is a no show or a last-minute cancellation.** Your usual reaction might be to just shrug and say, "Oh well."

But if you do the math and figure out how much money and time these lost appointments cost your practice, the number is staggering.

Let's say you personally produce $350 per hour and your hygienist generates $150 per hour. If you each lose just one appointment per day to no-shows and cancellations that's $500 per day x 4 days x 50 weeks = $100,000.00 per year down the drain!

I can't teach you how to *eliminate* all no-shows and last-minute cancellations... but I *can* train your team to cut them in *half*. That single Gem will boost your practice by no less than $50,000.00 per year (based upon just *one* no-show or last-minute cancellation per day for one doc and one RDH).

How to Add $100,000/Year in Cosmetic Dentistry
From Your Existing Patients
With Minimal Effort or Stress

GOLDMINE UNDERGROUND TEAM TRAINING TOOLKIT EPISODE 024

Do you enjoy performing cosmetic dentistry? As a Gems Platinum Family member one of the Team Training Toolkits you'll have at your fingertips will help you to identify and motivate existing patients... to the tune of $10,000 per month (or more) in cosmetic cases right under your nose that you're currently not even considering.

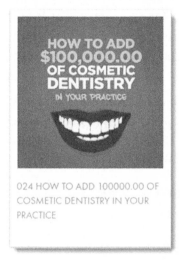

024 HOW TO ADD 100000.00 OF COSMETIC DENTISTRY IN YOUR PRACTICE

These are your existing happy patients who routinely come back time and again on recall but may never have voiced the slightest concern about the appearance of their smile. Of course, the last thing you'd want to do is offend a loyal happy patient by suggesting that she "fix" something *she* doesn't deem a problem.

During your **FREE 6-WEEK TEST DRIVE** of Gems Family Platinum membership, just ask your Personal Gems Concierge or Coach to point you to GoldMine Team Training Toolkit Episode 024, "How to Add $100,000.00 of Cosmetic Dentistry to Your Practice!" To claim your **FREE TEST DRIVE**, go to www.GemsAreEasy.com/Book5

TOBI MAKES GROWING YOUR PRACTICE EASY & STRESS-FREE

Perhaps the most far-reaching epiphany I experienced...

You don't need to use all the available Gems all at once. In fact, though counterintuitive... the more you try to do at once the *less* you'll succeed. Instead, your goal should be to find TOBI—The One Big Idea—and integrate it into your practice successfully. This philosophy isn't about increasing your workload. It's about finding points of leverage to decrease friction and waste, so you can help more people get well.

Imagine if you deployed just ONE or TWO of these Gems over the next three or four months. It would take *very* little time or effort. Yet what would that do for your patients? What would it do for your bank account? What would an extra $100,000.00 per year mean to you, your family and your practice?

Many of our Gems Family members have experienced *multiples* of that level of income growth. And for most of them, the first simple step was to take the **6-WEEK FREE TEST DRIVE** available at www.GemsAreEasy.com/Book5

A FEW LAST WORDS ABOUT THE GENERAL PRINCIPLES HERE...

Many patients refuse recommendations for getting the best possible care, saying that they don't have the time, or that it's too much money. But the TRUTH is that more often than not, they simply don't believe they really need the care you're offering. Or even if they "get" that what you're recommending is important, they don't see that their need is *urgent*.

With Gems on your side, it's possible to help many more patients realize the immediate benefits of what you're offering. *That's when they'll say yes* to your recommendations for maintaining their long-term health and happiness.

COLLECTIONS SOARED FROM
$650,000 PER YEAR TO $1,400,000!

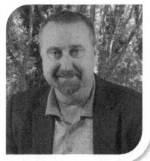

I was just not happy with what I was doing. I'd used dental consultants before. Paid a huge amount of money—and nothing changed. No forward movement. We actually went backwards. I was really jaded and had no appetite to sign with another consultant.

When I met Tom, he was a guest speaker at a dental meeting. His speech resonated with what I was going through. I could relate to the struggles he faced before he turned his practice around. At the time, I was on the verge of getting out of private practice altogether.

I chatted with Tom and shared my plans. He said, "Before you sell, why don't we assess where you're at?" Being a skeptic, I hesitated. But the fact that Tom is a dentist—one who had a compelling story that resonated with mine—opened my mind.

The rest is history. I abandoned my plan to sell. Three years ago, when I started with Tom, we were collecting $650,000 in annual revenue. **Today, we're collecting $1,400,000 yearly—more than double what we were before Gems!**

Tom got my team all rowing in the same direction. You can't do it without your crew. I had weekly phone calls with Wayne, my Personal Gems Concierge. If I had a question, I could email or call Wayne any time.

Soon we had instituted the Quadrant Challenge, which became one of our most successful Gems. The Quadrant Challenge involves breaking the mouth up into four parts during restorative treatment planning. Instead of just looking at one tooth at a time, you're working on the whole quadrant. You save your patients time, improve their overall health, and get their work done faster.

Our team understood the benefits of the Gem. With this Gem alone, we were well on our way to doubling our annual practice revenue.

We originally had a $5,000 daily goal. Now that number has doubled to $10,000 daily, and we often exceed even *that* amount. Before Gems, I couldn't conceive of doing $10,000 a day. But once you change *how* you're doing *what* you're doing, it's surprisingly easy. It only sounds crazy till you've done it for yourself.

If you told me before Gems that I'd be collecting close to $2 million a year, I would have said you were smoking crack, that there was no way I'd ever achieve that level of success.

But the reality is, we are *well* on our way to that new goal! Amazingly it's the small changes which have made a huge, huge difference. With Gems, the more people you help to achieve better health, the better you do.

I believe the key to my rebound has been using Tom's Gems—and working with his team. We've made major progress in short order.

—DR. KEN RASBORNIK, Cleveland, North Carolina

Want to discover exactly what Ken did so you can implement it in your practice? Take a **FREE 6-Week Test Drive** of my Gems Platinum Team Training Toolkit.

Go to www.GemsAreEasy.com/Book5

Long-Term Internal Financing

GOLDMINE UNDERGROUND TEAM TRAINING TOOLKIT EPISODE 015

What if you have a patient who wants to say yes to your recommended treatment but simply cannot proceed due to an inability to pay for it, even in two or three payments? What if this person is also unable to obtain third-party financing for the treatment?

If you let this patient leave without helping solve their problem, their oral health won't improve, and you're effectively saying no to more revenue. GoldMine Team Training Toolkit Episode 015, "Huge Profits Financing the Unfinanceable" can close this gap.

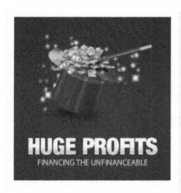

015 HUGE PROFITS · FINANCING THE UNFINANCEABLE

Affordable in-house extended payment plans for patients who can't afford your recommendations for care when offered short-term pay plans (patients who are turned down by your outside third-party financing companies).

With this Gem, I can almost hear you saying, *who in their right mind would assume that kind of risk?*

The answer: smart dentists who know how to choose the *right* candidates for this program, and a few key principles which help to mitigate that risk. Not only do these Gem-savvy dentists keep revenue from walking out the door—they generate additional (100% PURE PROFIT) revenue in return for the extended payment plan.

BUT WAIT... THERE'S MORE.

Can you see the possibilities here? Again, this is only a small handful of Gems, each of which can radically improve your revenue stream. But there are more Gems to discover.

A lot more.

How many?

Try 1000.

That's right. Over the years, I've identified at least *a thousand different Gems* that dentists can put to use to boost their revenue with very little effort.

YOU DON'T NEED ALL THE GEMS

I mentioned that there are at least 1000 Gems. But you don't need all of them—not even close. In fact, some of my most successful Gems Family Members have <u>grown their practice by millions of dollars by utilizing just 3 or 4 each year</u>!

But the fact is, *you don't actually need my help to find Gems.* They are out there to be discovered. You just have to know where to look and take the time and effort to see if the ones you find will really work for your practice.

That's pretty much how I discovered my Gems.

On the other hand, you don't *have* to become your own Gem hunter—unless of course you want to. I've already found and polished enough of these Gems to help us all add millions of dollars to our bottom line.

If you take advantage of my offer for a **6-week Free Test Drive of Gems Family Platinum membership**, you'll have access to all these Gems, off the shelf, and more. (For details go to www.GemsAreEasy.com/Book5)

And in the time it would take you to start from scratch, you'll already be witnessing a dramatic transformation in your practice. (I'll give you all the details on how you can do this at the end of this book.)

And you already have a few of these Gems in your hand, all ready to go! All you need is to take that first step...

Some Gems will make sense for your practice, and some won't. Some may interest you personally, and others may not. My best advice for making the most of these Gems is two-fold:

1. DEPLOY JUST ONE GEM AT A TIME.

Multi-tasking is a myth, anyway. Don't get overwhelmed by the field of Gems; just take the first one and make it work for you, then pick up another. (You'll also be better able to measure your results this way.)

2. CHOOSE THE GEMS THAT FIT YOU BEST.

Don't waste time or energy on a Gem just because it could get you more revenue and make your patients happier. All the Gems can do that. These Gems are designed to be easy to implement—no headaches. If a certain Gem doesn't fit your vision and workflow—just pick another one.

74

SHOULD I JUST CLOSE MY PRACTICE?

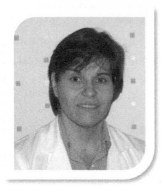

My practice was in crisis. We were in a rut. I was caring for a new baby, and we had a lot of overhead having built a new building for the practice. The culture of the practice wasn't vibrant. Our team gave good service, but we were stagnant.

I sat down with my husband for a hard talk. Should I close the practice and go work for someone else? We'd be rid of the overhead and the drama and the headaches. It was a tough decision because we weren't even sure that there was a way out.

I was near the end of my rope. But Tom seemed positive. I had heard many of the ideas he discussed in the past, but something about the way he presented them resonated with me. We decided to join the Gems Family and take a shot.

Immediately to turn things around we used a Gem called WHALYAs to motivate patients to get work they needed done sooner. We cranked on the WHALYAs. The patients loved them.

Another successful Gem was Elizabeth's Fractured Amalgam. This video empowered hygienists to motivate patients in need, to accept our recommendations for crowns. It generated lots of revenue. We've started doing same-day crowns, and patients love that.

Tom showed us how to find, negotiate with and hire in-house specialists, like an endodontist and periodontist. Instead of referring out this work, we kept it inside the practice. That brought in a big chunk of money, and patients love the convenience. They already know our staff, and having specialists right here saves them time.

We saw a big bump once we started working with Tom—easily an extra $300,000 in revenue. And we've sustained that growth over the years.

What's maybe even more exciting is what this process has done for the staff. They're so upbeat. We recently took them to one of Tom's masterminds. We all loved the masterminds—my husband still talks about them.

Gems motivated everybody. What's amazing, looking back, is that we didn't have to change that many things to see revenue growth and refresh our team's culture. It was surprisingly simple!

—*DR. MARY ANN GARCIA, Raynham, Massachusetts*

Want to experience a transformation like Dr. Garcia? The first step is to take a **FREE 6-Week Test Drive** of my Gems Platinum Team Training Toolkit.

Go to www.GemsAreEasy.com/Book5

CHAPTER 6

THE INCREDIBLE JOURNEY OF DR. KELLY BROWN

You're now familiar with the Gems philosophy and why it works. And now you've had a chance to see how Gems have been used by some of our colleagues as well. Hopefully, you're already testing out one or more of the Gems I've already shared with you, and you're seeing results. Now, I want to share a story that will show you just how much potential these Gems carry.

It is with great privilege that I share with you the story of Dr. Kelly Brown, in his own words. His story encompasses profound tragedy and success. I hope it ties together the lessons we've presented in this book and reinforces themes that I think are profoundly powerful.

"How Tom's Gems Helped Me Vault from $1.3 Million and No Retirement in Sight To $17,000,000.00 per Year!"

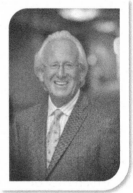

I'm Dr. Kelly Brown, dentist and founder of Custom Dental in Edmond, Oklahoma.

I landed in this field by default. I started out at OU College in engineering, then decided to become a zoologist. Later that year, I met the love of my life, my wife, Jan. And she asked a really good question: "What are you going to do with a zoology degree? Have you ever thought about medicine or something like that?"

I looked at what was happening to most of the zoology graduates. They were usually graduating, getting a shovel, and getting asked to follow the south end of a northbound elephant. I was not interested in that. I grew up in a small town. We had a dentist. We had a physician. I looked at their lifestyle. It was an easy choice. I decided at that point I would be a dentist, and I've never regretted it.

Well-Intentioned Bad Advice

When I first started out, though, I got some really bad advice.

I kind of halfway knew how to fix teeth, but I had no idea on how to set up a business. I told a professor at the dental school, "I'm going back to my hometown. So, what do I do?"

He said, "Well, Kelly, it's simple. You just go to your town and see what everybody else is doing. What hours are they open? What procedures are they offering? What fees are they charging? *Just do what they do, and you'll be okay.*"

What, exactly, does "okay" mean? In my case, apparently, it meant starving. For the first two years, I couldn't even bring home a paycheck. Thank God my wife was gainfully employed, but I was in total frustration.

I went on like that for almost a decade, and I looked for all kinds of options to escape. If there would have been an easy door out, I would have left.

Trapped. Broke. Jammed.

I think in part because of that bad advice I'd received, my perception of what a dental practice should be was totally distorted. This caused all kinds of challenges. My staff was apathetic. They were clock punchers, but I had no leadership skills and no vision other than getting out of this hole. As a result, we were drawing patients who were not happy with the practice. I hated that. In truth, there wasn't one thing I liked about my practice. Financially, I was jammed. I was in my own small hometown. I couldn't just dump everything and tell everybody, "I'm sorry I owe you money, but we're done." I had to show up every day to try and make good to them. I really wasn't doing anything for me. I was just trapped.

Then the Worst Thing Happened

One day, while I was at my office, I got the worst phone call anybody could ever get. They said, "Dr. Brown, your two-year-old son has been in an accident, and we're rushing him to the hospital." I really don't know what happened for the next 30 minutes, other than I was out of the office and at the hospital. They med-flighted him to Oklahoma City, where he was pronounced dead.

Not only was I crushed emotionally, I was also embarrassed financially. We already had too many credit cards loaded with debt, and here I was going to have to take out another one. *I had to borrow money to bury my son.*

I remember heading back to the office a week later. I was sickened, with this fist-in-the-stomach kind of feeling you just can't get away from. I knew I was going to be greeted by unhappy patients, because

I'd been gone a week; an apathetic staff, because they didn't really care; and a stack of unpayable bills on my desk.

That'll Never Work Here

Shortly after my return to the office I left, again, to attend a seminar. I came back all excited. I told my staff about the changes we were going to make—and they all quit. They reacted like, "No, Dr. Brown, not you, not in this town. That'll never work."

It was actually a good thing because it gave me an opportunity to bring in people who could *believe* in my dream at that moment. The new people I hired didn't know the old stories, so within a short period of time, I went from having a low-producing dental practice to a fairly nice practice.

But I still was stuck with a problem. I had feared that I would reach retirement age without being able to retire financially stress-free. I was making good money when I was working, but I was losing money whenever I left the office. My new mindset had helped stabilize my practice, but it wasn't enough. I still couldn't plan for the future.

Add $60,000.00 to Your Bottom Line. Tomorrow.

After trying a few different things without much success, I received an envelope in the mail. It contained a CD from this crazy Gems guy named Tom with a promise on the CD title: "Add $60,000 to your bottom line tomorrow." I remember thinking, *either this guy's nuts, or he's got something.*

I listened to the CD, <u>I used one of his Gems, and lo and behold, I added $60,000 to my bottom line</u>. This was before I'd ever met him, become a member, or anything else.

That made me a believer.

I decided I needed to meet this Tom guy in person, so later that year, I went to his Gems Family Retreat in Boston. When I connected with Tom and his group, I felt like I'd finally found a place of likeminded people. I had reached outside my industry for answers, but prior to Gems, I had never been in a room of dentists who felt and thought the same way I did.

I felt like I was home.

From then on, nothing was the same. I saw a path and a support system that could make my dream possible. From late summer 2006 to October 2008, I went from one practice to a second; eventually, we had four practices. And at that point, because of the Gems I had learned from Tom, I transformed my income and my career. I stopped being a swapping-hours-for-dollars dentist and became a business owner.

Pick and Choose from a Buffet of Gems

When I walked into Tom's world, I realized that Tom had created a dental management buffet. He says there are 1000 Gems, but there may be more than 1000. And they're all accessible to any dentist who is part of his operation. Of course, I've not loaded more than a handful of his 1000 Gems on my plate, but the ones I have discovered and used have changed my life remarkably.

I chose to withdraw from patient care in October of 2008, and from then on, I spent my time working on the business side of my practice. I also began spending more time with my wife and enjoying the fruits of the labor that we had put together.

Fast-forward 10 years. We now have 16 practices in four states. Last year, we did $17 million as an organization. We brought 7,000 new patients into our organization. We have a huge patient base, and we're touching a lot of lives in a lot of communities.

Thanks to Tom's help, I've been able to develop a dream team and a dental machine that enables me to run it with about 15 hours a week of my time. That leaves me time for my family and time to volunteer in my community. I live in an exclusive gated golf community, so I sneak off and play golf anytime I want.

I don't have an office to show up to. The only traffic jam I deal with is at the coffeepot with Jan in the morning.

Jan and I love to spend time with our grandchildren, and we have plenty of opportunities to do that. One of our passions is travel, so we make sure we travel approximately a week every month. This year, we've been to Tahiti, the Amalfi Coast in Italy, Sicily, Denmark and Holland.

I make more in a month than many dentists do in a year. Thanks to Gems, I'm now living my dream of a financially stress-free retirement.

—DR. KELLY BROWN, Guthrie, Oklahoma

Stories like these drive me to do what I do.
I would be honored to help you create the
practice of your dreams too.
The very first step is to take a
FREE 6-Week Test Drive of my
Gems Platinum Team Training Toolkit.

Go to www.GemsAreEasy.com/Book5

CHAPTER 7

LOOKING BACK ON OUR JOURNEY

We've raced through a tremendous amount in a relatively short book. I want to personally thank you for taking the time to engage energetically with this material.

It takes courage to explore unfamiliar ideas. Many dentists are less than happy with their status quo yet will sadly never escape it. And that's tragic.

Operating from the wrong mental model limits your ability to help your patients achieve maximum health and longevity, limits your ability to create a more ideal workplace for your team, and constrains your ability to make use of your natural gifts. Fear and inertia impact the world at large.

So many dentists labor and struggle; they're doing the same activities they've done for years, hoping for different results. They've never questioned mistaken ideas about how to run a practice—beliefs that have been transmitted to them by the culture or handed down by well-meaning but misguided colleagues.

The key to unlocking the potential of your practice is not grit, nor burning the midnight oil, nor suffering. It's about restructuring a few beliefs about what it takes to succeed, both in business and in life.

Gems teach leverage. Make small strategic tweaks to your operation, then see them through with solid execution, support, and coaching. This is the way to create positive, lasting change.

You now hold in your hand a few battle-tested Gems: WHALYAs, the Fluoride Verbal Skills, and my Theory of the Bobble-Headed Dog. Put them into practice. I want you to see what you can do. I want your world to be better for having read this book.

There's no need to move mountains just to extract coal. The riches you seek are all around you, Gems glittering in the sun. All you need to do is look around, and simply pick them up.

CHAPTER 8

THE ROAD AHEAD

You understand the Gems philosophy. Now you're at a crossroads. There are several possible paths ahead. I can't tell you which one to go down.

Path #1. You close this book, forget you ever read it, and go back to business as usual.

Maybe your intuition is better than mine. Maybe you'll derive your own tactics and leverage. Maybe a DIY approach will lead you to overcome the obstacles and frustrations that are painfully familiar. If this is your choice, I hope it does.

Path #2: You take the information in this book and deploy it in your practice just to see what happens.

Perhaps you will test out the Fluoride Verbal Skills Gem, WHALYAs and/or The Bobble-Headed Dog and drive up your annual income as you help your patients receive treatment that will make them healthier. I will consider this book a success if it motivated you to do just that. But I want more for you than that...

Path #3: Galvanized to make change, you and I continue to work together... So, the question you may be wondering is HOW do we make this happen?

The fastest and by far the EASIEST way is to **allow me to continue to help you... for FREE**.

www.GemsAreEasy.com/Book5

Let me tell you how I'm going to do that. The opportunity to grow your revenue and your personal net income is enormous.

My team and I will help train *your* team on WHALYAs and Adult Fluoride. Deployed effectively, you could easily enjoy a $50,000 to $100,000 increase *just* from those two Gems. And while that $50,000 to $100,000 you're currently leaving on the table may seem like a lot of money, there's a LOT more...

It's just the tip of the tip of the iceberg. In fact, the <u>average general dentist is missing out on AT LEAST $250,000 per year</u>.

We'll train your team, for FREE,
on those two Gems and a *lot* more.
Take advantage of my offer of a
6-WEEK FREE TEST-DRIVE
of **Gems Family Platinum membership.**

In addition to getting instant access to the online and team training by phone and screen share, I'll also be sending you a TREASURE CHEST (literally) of profit-producing Gems in the mail. I'll tell you more about that in a minute.

Gems Platinum is normally $497 a month. But if you take the **SIX-WEEK FREE TEST-DRIVE**, initially you'll only be charged a one-time shipping fee of $6. Your card will not be charged the $497 monthly fee until week 7. Gems Family Platinum membership is month-to-month. You may cancel at any time.

Although there is no obligation to continue working with me after your 6-week FREE trial, if you're like most dentists, not continuing your membership would be unthinkable. But don't decide now if this is for you. Just take the 6-Week FREE Test Drive and experience the results of being a Gems Family Platinum member.

Go RIGHT NOW to **www.GemsAreEasy.com/Book5** to take advantage of this FREE offer, and you'll receive...

Easy Gem #1:

"Adult Fluoride, Add $50,000/Year, per RDH!"

GoldMine UnderGround Team Training Toolkit Episode 051

This Gems Team Training Toolkit includes the 4 Heavy Plastic Fluoride Verbal Skills 3 x 5 "Cheat Sheet" cards, and a VIDEO TEAM TRAINING by yours truly.

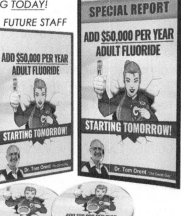

EASY GEM #1

ADD $40,000.00/YEAR, PER RDH, IN ADULT FLUORIDE! LEARN IN JUST 40 MINUTES TODAY. START USING TOMORROW!

- ONLINE VIDEO - INSTANT TEAM TRAINING *TODAY!*
- DVD VIDEO - TODAY, & WHEN ADDING FUTURE STAFF
- AUDIO MP3 - LISTEN ON THE GO!
- SPECIAL REPORT - UNEDITED UNABRIDGED TRANSCRIPT

I'll show you the research and share my simple verbal skills to help your hygienist convey to your adult patients exactly why adult Fluoride treatment following prophy is a critical piece of the maximum health puzzle... and with the help of this 60-second verbal skill, adults will **never again ask** **"Does my insurance cover it?"**

Instead, they'll **willingly and consistently accept and pay out of pocket for Fluoride!**

EASY GEM #2:

"SIX KEYS UNLOCK THE SECRET TO ADDING $100,000.00 / YEAR, PERIODONTAL PHASE I!"

GoldMine UnderGround Team Training Toolkit Episode 052

This Gems Team Training Toolkit includes the VIDEO TEAM TRAINING and a jaw-dropping laminated graphic which, when used with the verbal skills in the training, will help you help your patients perceive the immediate need for periodontal Phase One care, even in the absence of symptoms.

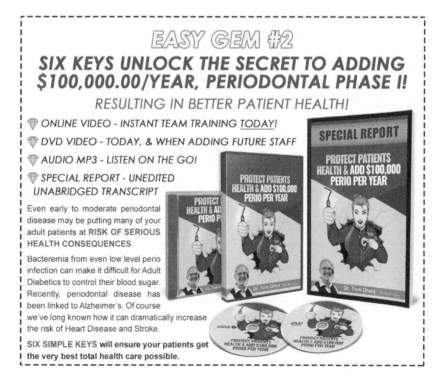

Easy Gem #3:

"A Team Bonus System that Works!"

GoldMine UnderGround Team Training Toolkit Episode 046

Not only will you get my VIDEO TEAM TRAINING TOOLKIT, we'll also supply you with our proprietary Team Bonus System Calculator... totally DONE-FOR-YOU, so you won't have to figure out a thing!

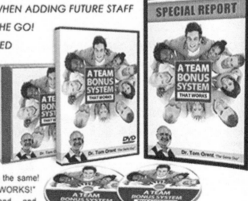

I Started Seeing Results Literally in the First Two Days!

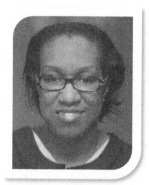

When I joined Tom's Gems Family, I was about 6 ½ months pregnant. I had a lot going on and wanted to get my practice stabilized and on a good path. I wanted to stabilize my staff, grow my practice and put systems in place to help me excel my practice and my life.

Tom's team bonus system is great.

It helps motivate everybody. Even in a practice that might have some slightly reluctant team members, **once they see Tom's Team Bonus System they actually want to get on board and do whatever it takes.** His program helps keep everyone accountable.

Tom provides a wealth of knowledge. The biggest benefit from Gems has been the growth of the practice. I started seeing results literally in the first two days. It took no time at all!

The most pleasant surprise is the caring, sharing and openness of the other Gems doctors. So often at dental society meetings or study clubs everyone's cordial, but without really meaning it. Gems members are truly genuine. They open their hearts and really want you to succeed.

You Are Not Alone

The best part of Gems is that you're not alone. There is always someone you can talk to, you can email, you can send out an email blast to other members via the Gems forum. Maybe you're in a predicament with staff or with a patient so you get input from the other members, or you can ask Tom or the Gems coaches. Plus, my Personal Gems Concierge is always available to help.

Accountability is key to success. My Gems Concierge makes me get off my butt and do what I need to do!

Life Transforming

Tom's program is the ultimate way to get things accomplished. Joining the program has given me the confidence to do the things I needed to do in my practice. It's my livelihood, it's how I plan on taking care of my kid and plan on having my retirement. It's my life and I have to step up to the plate. Tom has given me the confidence and tools to do it. It's transformative.

I don't feel like I have to worry anymore and that's a wonderful peace of mind. My priorities are my child, my family and my practice. I no longer have to worry my child will be okay. Whatever I need to provide for him, I'll be able to do it.

Since starting the program, I feel less stress at work. With all the different training Tom provides for your team, it helps make the day-to-day easier, which makes for a happy me!

If you are pondering whether Gems is the right choice for you, stop thinking about it. Join the family. You will be given all the tools you need to change your life. Gems is unlike any other program you've ever encountered. A wealth of knowledge, a wealth of camaraderie, a wealth of friendship and it helps you improve your practice.

—Dr. Erika Burley, Charlotte, North Carolina

Yes, you too could start seeing results
in your bank account in just two days.
Put my gems to the test for free.
Get your **6-Week FREE TEST DRIVE** here:

www.GemsAreEasy.com/Book5

1-888-880-GEMS (4367)

HIGHEST MONTH'S COLLECTIONS IN ALL MY YEARS PRACTICING!

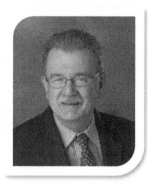

We made Team Bonus Goal last month (again!). It was the highest monthly collections we've ever recorded in all my years practicing!

And this month has started out with a bang as well. We've had production numbers of (cue the drum roll, fireworks and marching band!) Monday $31,990 and Wednesday $22,786. Not bad for a solo doc, eh?!

Before we started with Gems we were heavily in debt—particularly after investing in failed consulting forays with companies I will not mention here, but you would immediately recognize them if I did. Our equipment was antiquated and run-down, left as a legacy from the previous owner, and we were referring all our CBCTs to another office for our implant cases.

Now, just 18 months later we have:

1. **Paid off all our notes and credit card debt** that we accrued enlisting in non-productive marketing and consulting schemes.

2. **Upgraded our handpieces to electric**, eliminating ongoing costs for continual repairs to the old air rotors, and...

3. **Purchased a CBCT**, which allows us to keep our implant patients in-house and provide them with a WOW factor which has enabled us to close more cases and generate income over and above the monthly payment, thus turning our radiology department into a new profit center.

I realize that none of these are as glamorous as a boat, a new house or a sports car, but they are making or saving us a TON of MONEY, making us more efficient and tremendously profitable!

—*DR. AL ST. GERMAINE, Nashua, New Hampshire*

EASY GEM #4:

"HOW TO DOUBLE HYGIENE RECALL!"

GoldMine UnderGround Team Training Toolkit Episode 009

This may be *the* most popular Team Training Toolkit we've ever launched. Though you may not *double* hygiene recall, many of our Gems Family members *have* added at least a full day, often two... by deploying this one simple Gem!

Hygiene is the *engine* that drives a dental practice. Adding just 8 hours of hygiene per week often results in excess of a $200,000 increase in revenue ($70,000 from hygiene and $130,000+ from restorative diagnosed during recall exams).

EASY GEM #4
"HOW TO DOUBLE HYGIENE RECALL"

COULD BE THE EASIEST TO DEPLOY MOST IMPORTANT PROFIT-DRIVING DISCOVERY YOU MAKE FOR MANY YEARS TO COME

- 💎 *ONLINE VIDEO - INSTANT TEAM TRAINING TODAY!*
- 💎 *DVD VIDEO - TODAY, & WHEN ADDING FUTURE STAFF*
- 💎 *AUDIO MP3 - LISTEN ON THE GO!*
- 💎 *SPECIAL REPORT - UNEDITED UNABRIDGED TRANSCRIPT*

You probably will **NOT DOUBLE** your hygiene recall numbers using this little "Gem." That said, it wouldn't be at all unusual if you were able to **ADD ONE OR TWO ADDITIONAL FULL DAYS OF HYGIENE** to your schedule! And that's *per* doctor. If you are a two doctor practice, "How to Double Hygiene Recall" could add 2 or 3, even 4 days of jammed-packed hygiene appointments week in and week out from now until the day you retire. This Team Training Toolkit consists of TWO DIFFERENT proven effective strategies. Use just one, or use them both for results you can take to the bank!

"HYGIENE PROFITABILITY SHOT THROUGH THE ROOF! OUR PRACTICE IS UP A WHOPPING $303,948!!!"

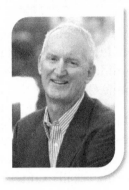

Tom, please share this with our colleagues who may have been through other programs.

I'd HAD "consultants" before, and I was hesitant that I was in for the same ol' same old.

One major well-known program kept saying if you throw in enough "closes," they're bound to say yes at some point! I also warned you that one of my hygienists, Pam, might not like my getting into another program. **She really didn't like the idea of Fluoride for adults**. 'Course I didn't agree with her one bit. I respected her right to her professional opinion, but I didn't know how to help her understand the critical benefits, especially for adults.

Your helping Pam broaden her professional understanding of the rationale for appropriate top-notch treatment has improved the level of excellent care our patients now enjoy.

That alone is wonderful, but the PROFITABILITY of my HYGIENE DEPARTMENT LITERALLY SHOT THROUGH THE ROOF!

My two RDH's are up a combined annualized total of $124,920! Our patients are getting THE best care, and our hygiene department is SUPER-PROFITABLE!

But the VERY best news is that our entire office is up a whopping annualized $303,948!!!

I wanted Gems to help not only my family and me, not just my patients, but I truly want to share more with my wonderful team.

Thanks to you I have been able to pay EVERY staff member over $2,000.00 in BONUSES in just the last 6 months!

Gems is unlike ANY other program out there. You have combined a powerful mixture of so much great, but SIMPLE TO IMPLEMENT information, my team and I will be forever grateful for inviting us into your program.

Thanks, from the bottom of our hearts.

—*DR. JOE ALBERT, Edmonds, Washington*

Want to skyrocket your hygiene profitability like Dr. Albert? It's easy. Simply go to

www.GemsAreEasy.com/Book5 and start your **FREE 6-Week Test Drive**.

After you go to www.GemsAreEasy.com/Book5 and read about Gems Family Platinum, click on "JOIN PLATINUM." The usual $497/month will be WAIVED for your first 6 weeks. You'll be asked only to pay a one-time $6 fee for shipping. Your credit card will not be charged the usual $497/month until your 7th week. You may cancel at any time.

In the 4 Easy Gem Team Training modules, you'll get access to team video toolkits I filmed, which will help you and inspire your team to achieve measurably increased case acceptance of best-option care.

In the Easy Gem #1 video training I help your team understand *why* Fluoride is so important for adults. I take them step-by-step, hand-in-hand sharing additional powerful tools to help you persuade your adult patients of the *need* for and benefits of Fluoride treatment. Using my Simple Seven Sentence Script, as many as 80% of your adult patients will happily pay out of pocket for Fluoride.

The Video TEAM TRAINING TOOLKIT will help your team practice and role play and ramp up to speed with the highest possible acceptance as quickly as possible.

Remember, I've shared my Fluoride verbal skills with you earlier in the book. I encourage you to deploy them and see for yourself!

When you sign up for the **6-WEEK FREE TEST DRIVE**, you'll also receive a new member welcome package, a (literal) TREASURE CHEST overflowing with lots of fun things— including surprises that your team will love. This package contains 4 heavy plastic 3 x 5 Fluoride Verbal Skills cards. So whenever new team members come onboard, you can train them easily. These heavy-duty 3 x 5 "cheat sheet" verbal skills cards will keep your team sharp and at peak performance.

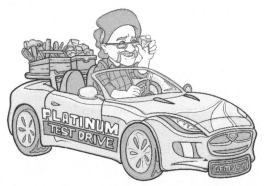

FREE TEST DRIVE GEMS FAMILY PLATINUM

As a Gems Family member, you'll be assigned a Personal Gems Concierge. Your Gems Concierge will be available to help you find and deploy a wide range of Gems resources available to Gems Family Platinum members. You also get a 30-minute call with one of our coaches. During this call, your coach will help your team get comfortable with the Fluoride Verbal Skills and answer any questions.

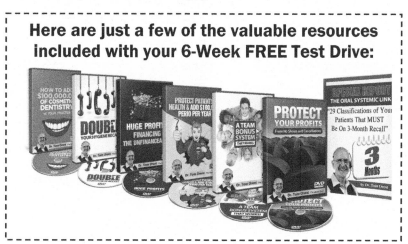

Here are just a few of the valuable resources included with your 6-Week FREE Test Drive:

- Gems Perio protocol and verbal skills: "7 Steps to Ensure Increased Acceptance of Periodontal Phase I Care"
- "Team Bonus System 2.0" including a DONE-FOR-YOU Team Bonus System Calculator.
- "How to Double Hygiene Recall"
- Special Report, "The Oral Systemic Link: 29 Classifications of Adult Patients Who Must Be on More Frequent Recall."
- "Protect Your Profits from No-Shows & Last-Minute Cancellations"
- "How to Add $100,000/Year in Cosmetic Dentistry from Your Existing Patients with Minimal Effort or Stress"
- Long-Term Internal Financing Gem, "Financing the Unfinanceable!"

These bonuses are all available for free (for the first 97 dentists who respond) at **www.GemsAreEasy.com/Book5**. But I want to emphasize again that you don't need the bonuses in order to start making money and helping more patients—right now. So, get testing!

"ONE DOC. SMALL TEAM. BIG INCREASE OF $430,204.00!"

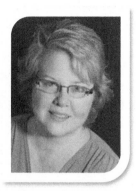

Tom starts with what he calls **"The low hanging fruit"**—easy techniques that really make a big difference in the health of your patients and your practice!

I have a very small practice. It's just me, one assistant and a front desk person. Before Gems my practice was losing patients. My town has had ZERO growth for six years now and my efforts to get patients weren't working.

Before I joined Gems, my practice was very stressful. I felt like I was putting in all this time and nothing was happening. But thanks to Tom and Gems I'm back to loving dentistry again!

I love the fact that Gems is provided by someone who was in the trenches. **It took just two weeks for me to see our production double!**

What I didn't like about other consulting firms was that they asked me to do things that I didn't feel were in the patient's best interest. With Gems you get to pick things that make sense to you from the hundreds of things they offer. Choose a half-dozen or so strategies you like and your practice skyrockets!

After just two weeks my team was so excited when they saw how much we'd improved without that much effort. They love it!

Gaining Acceptance of the Very Best Possible Care

In our hearts we know what our patients need. We want them to have and accept the treatment we recommend. Now, having the right words gives me confidence.

We're having more fun. There's more joy in every day.

It only took 90 minutes to implement our very first Gem. We started applying it right away and in just two weeks we had a huge bump. It really didn't take much at all!

If you're considering joining our Gems Family, just do it. I can't imagine not having joined Gems. It's been such a huge life changer.

It makes such a difference when your team is 110% behind you in a way that really supports the practice. Once they take an ownership mentality, they're going to love it... and you're going to explode with happiness. Your practice will just skyrocket. I never expected to do this well this quickly. Tom's program has changed my life.

Just one doc and a small team... but thanks to Gems, in just 10 months, a BIG INCREASE of $430,204.00!

—DR. TERRIE CRIBBS, Knoxville, Tennessee

Gems are EASY and they can help you enjoy a profound personal and professional transformation.

Go to www.GemsAreEasy.com/Book5 to take advantage of your **6-Week FREE TEST DRIVE** of Gems Family Platinum membership. Just click on "JOIN PLATINUM."

There's actually a *lot* more available to you as a Gems Family Platinum member...

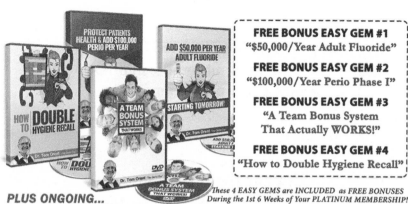

PLUS ONGOING...

- ✓ ADVANCED MARKETING BRAIN TRUST
- ✓ COMPUTER ENHANCED **SMILE IMAGING**
- ✓ CUSTOM DESIGN & PERSONALIZED NEW PATIENT MUGS
- ✓ PERSONAL TEAM TRAINING **COACHING CALLS**
- ✓ **COACHING CALLS** WITH ELIZABETH ORENT "ENGINEER"
- ✓ RAPID RESPONSE EMERGENCY **PHONE CONSULTATIONS**
- ✓ ADVERTISEMENT CRITIQUES
- ✓ GROUP MASTERMIND MEETINGS, LIVE VIA THE WEB
- ✓ GOLDRUSH PATIENT MOTIVATION DONE-FOR-YOU PROFIT SYSTEMS
- ✓ CUSTOMIZED GOLDRUSH PATIENT MOTIVATOR BUTTONS
- ✓ PRACTICE CALENDAR DESIGN
- ✓ MASTERMIND RETREATS - SPRING & FALL LIVE EVENTS
- ✓ ASK DR. TOM MEMBER-ONLY 90-MINUTE Q & A NIGHTS
- ✓ **GOLDMINE UNDERGROUND TEAM TRAINING TOOLKITS**
- ✓ "FRACTURED!" C&B CASE PRESENTATION STORYBOARD
- ✓ GEMS INSIDERS' CIRCLE WEBINARS
- ✓ NEW FRONTIERS DENTAL PRACTICE SUCCESS NEWSLETTER

I hope you enjoyed and will *profit* from reading this book. I always love feedback. If you have any questions or suggestions, I'd love to hear from you. You can email me at Tom@1000Gems.com

Remember, you're only one Gem away!

**"A year from now you'll
wish you had started today!"**
Karen Lamb

MORE FROM OUR COLLEAGUES ABOUT DR. TOM ORENT'S "GEMS"

"I used to do one crown at a time, or sometimes even a very large MODBL composite. Gems method of presenting quadrant dentistry has really skyrocketed our practice. The confidence and increase in revenue that you get from Gems literally is a life changer. We went from $600,000 to $1,000,000 in just 10 months. I just bought a Mercedes and a summer place on a West Hampton Beach. Going with Tom and Elizabeth was one of the best decisions I ever made."

—DR. GEORGE LANDRESS, Danbury, Connecticut

"I'm writing this from my NEW SKI CHALET at Mt. Snow that I bought with the extra cash as a result of Tom's program... after stashing away a BIG CHUNK to retirement."

—DR. DOUG BLACKMORE, Ramsey, New Jersey

"Thanks to Gems, I have more personal freedom now than ever before."

—DR. STEVE ABEL, Mount Kisco, New York

"I've taken a TON of advanced continuing education—Pankey through level IV, LVI anterior and posterior functional esthetics, and a one-year implant residency... all of which were incredible yet... none of them came anywhere close to teaching you how to get patients to ACCEPT that kind of care. Tom and the Gems Team have exceeded anything I could have hoped for. They taught us how to get patients to accept very best care. Now we're up $238,836 in just 9 months with Gems!"

—DR. DEBORAH MANOS, Grosse Pointe Woods, Michigan

"Tom, we have tripled new patient flow and increased collections by $402,444 in 9 months. But this is NOT the most important part of what you've done for us! Thanks to Gems our family now has a practice whose strength will take it into the 2nd generation of Jenkins' doctors."

—DR. ALVIN AND CAROLYN JENKINS
West Jefferson, North Carolina

"In just 5 or 6 weeks we'd implemented some of the easy low-hanging fruit Gems. The gains come right away. Many of Tom's concepts can be done easily with little effort. Tom puts his heart and soul into what he's doing. We're up $378,682 in 10 months!"

—*DR. JONATHAN GLATT, Lakewood, New Jersey*

"The part of the Gems program that's made the biggest impact has been the chance to brainstorm with business minds about questions we have regarding growing to the next level. It almost doesn't matter which of Tom's Gems you try first as long as you try something. Since joining Gems our revenue has increased 22% over last year."

—*DR. GARY LOGIN, Brookline, Massachusetts*

"Before Gems I thought I faced possibly insurmountable odds. I was a young doctor in an area of well-established older practices. Our local population chooses a dentist mainly based on their PPO insurance. But after less than a year with Gems, new patient exams have increased 43%, I'm able to reward my incredible team, and our revenue is up $277,704! From the bottom of my heart, thank you, Tom and Elizabeth."

—*DR. JEFF LAFURIA, Warren, Ohio*

"In the first year, our revenue went up 25%."

—*DR. MAT ARONOFF, New York, New York*

"I started seeing results literally in the first 2 days! It took no time at all! Tom's Team Bonus System helps motivate Everybody. Tom's program has transformed my life."

—*DR. ERIKA BURLEY, Charlotte, North Carolina*

"I've gone from hating work to bouncing out of bed eager to see what new and fun things we can find to do with our patients in less than a year. My small town didn't seem capable of supporting the type of practice I wanted... and now we're up $239,512!"

—*DR. JEFFREY GOLDSTEIN, Penndel, Pennsylvania*

"Thinking I needed a consultant on-site in-office was a fallacy. Tom and his team were spot on with everything. We've gone from 50% case acceptance to right around 80%. Gems has changed every facet of my life. It's the greatest decision I've ever made."

—DR. DORIAN HAMPTON, Carrollton, Texas

"Tom's Team Bonus System had a big impact—immediately brought everyone on board and for the first time they really had a personal stake in the health of the practice."

—DR. PAUL BOOKMAN, Bryn Mawr, Pennsylvania

"Since joining Gems I have less stress and more free time... and that's what life is all about. After joining Gems, we started seeing benefits in less than 2 weeks!"

—DR. KENNETH BLACK, Chapel Hill, North Carolina

"Like a lot of doctors, I've spent most of my time attempting to be a better clinical dentist and failed to put as much effort or time into the business and marketing end of my practice as I should have. I used to have a hard time getting patients to understand and perceive the need for treatment. The way Tom taught us to present treatment, his deep and accurate insight into how patients would accept our highest recommendations, is the greatest gift Tom gave us. Net revenues are up over 35%."

—DR. KEVIN MAHONEY
Fellow of the American Dental Soc. of Anesthesiology
Erie, Pennsylvania

"Prior to Gems a good month was $40,000.00. Today I collect at least $130,000.00 a month! Tom's Gems program has changed my life. We were able to build the home of our dreams and financed our house for only 10 years. Our team members are excited to come to work. They know they make a big difference in the practice. They're happy and that translates into happy patients!"

—DR. MIKE MCKINNEY, Prestonsburg, Kentucky

FREE AUDIO BOOK "CoalMine to GoldMine!"
www.CoaltoGold.com/AUDIOBOOK

FREE VERBAL SKILLS TOOLKIT proven to help patients achieve better health and increase your practice revenue by as much as $40,000 to $50,000! **www.CoaltoGold.com/AUDIOBOOK**

THREE FREE TEAM TRAINING VIDEOS www.GemsAreEasy.com/VIDEOS

1. BOBBLE-HEADED DOG ACHIEVES MAXIMUM CASE ACCEPTANCE!

95% of the problems we diagnose and treat are ones we recommend in the *absence* of symptoms. YOUR PATIENTS WILL TRUST YOUR HYGIENIST MORE than they trust you. When your hygienist is *first* to mention the need for care in the absence of symptoms, and you follow as a second opinion *confirming* what she already stated, YOUR CASE ACCEPTANCE AND PRACTICE REVENUE WILL INCREASE!

2. ADD $50,000/YEAR WITH ADULT FLUORIDE.

Be my guest and watch the same step-by-step detailed VIDEO TEAM TRAINING TOOLKIT my Gems Family members enjoy. In this video I'll train your team on the rationale—the *necessity* behind offering Fluoride to every adult. My explanation in this video *plus* the Seven Simple Sentence Verbal Skills will *ensure* your highest possible adult patient acceptance of Fluoride... and nearly $50,000 increase in annual revenue per RDH.

3. ADD $100,000 PER YEAR WITH WHALYAs.

If you added just *one* small WHALYA each day, e.g. $400, you've just increased your revenue by $2,000 per week and $100,000 per year! We've just barely scratched the surface of how to most effectively deploy WHALYAs in your practice. This Video Team Training Toolkit on WHALYAs will get you up and running in *less* than 1 hour... trained *and* ready to deploy!

FREE 6-WEEK TEST DRIVE
OF GEMS FAMILY PLATINUM

Go to **www.GemsAreEasy.com/Book5** and read about Gems Family Platinum, then click on "JOIN PLATINUM." The usual $497/month will be WAIVED for your first 6 weeks. You'll be asked only to pay a one-time $6 fee for shipping. Your credit card will not be charged the usual $497/month until your 7th week. You may cancel at any time. This is only a fraction of what you'll get during your FREE TEST DRIVE.

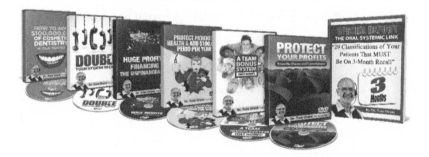

Wouldn't It Be Nice to **Have Someone Else Train Your Team** on How to Consistently Get 80% of Your Patients to Accept a Highly Beneficial Treatment You're Rarely If Ever Offering…

"Reserve Your FREE 30-Minute Team Training Call To Enable Your Patients to Achieve Better Health & Boost Your Revenue by $50,000 per RDH…"

Without Spending 1 More on Advertising

So Why Did We Give Up Offering Fluoride to Adults?

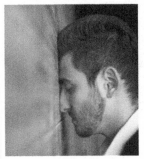

The reason most of our colleagues no longer offer Fluoride to adults is because we fear the inevitable response:

"Will My Insurance Cover That?"

The more I researched the rationale for giving Fluoride to adults, and the more I learned about the potential negative consequences of NOT giving Fluoride to adults, the more I realized I had an ethical responsibility to my adult patients when it came to Fluoride. I had a responsibility to ensure that I did everything ethically possible to make certain that they not only understood the need but were willing to accept the recommendation… even though they must pay out-of-pocket, because insurance won't cover Fluoride for adults.

The challenge therefore is that even though topical Fluoride treatment at the end of the prophy visit may be even MORE important for adults than it is for children, few know how to convey it to patients in a proven, effective manner.

Reserve your FREE 30-minute, live one-on-one team training phone call…

…and your team will discover how, in just seven sentences, you can achieve 80% (or better) acceptance of Fluoride by adults, who will gladly pay for the treatment out of pocket. Here are the results from just a few of the hundreds of hygienists who've gone through our 30-minute training:

Doctor	RDH	Adult Fluoride Paid Out-of-Pocket
Dr. Kirstin Ramsay	Suzanne	100%
Dr. Bill Gioia	Kim	100%
Dr. Michael Alsouss	Gabrielle	92%
&	Jamal	93%
Dr. Bob Dernick	Brandie	100%
Dr. David Hanle	Nicole	88%
Dr. Ike Lans	Michelle	90%
Dr. Anna Pollatos	Nancy	89%
Dr. Jerry Rinehart	Kim	100%

Reserve your FREE 30-Min. Live One-on-One Team Training Call TODAY!

Go to www.7SimpleSentences.com/BOOK5